SpringerBriefs in Well-Being and Quality of Life Research

D1825076

For further volumes:
http://www.springer.com/series/10150

Silvia Exenberger · Barbara Juen

Well-Being, Resilience and Quality of Life from Children's Perspectives

A Contextualized Approach

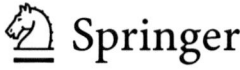 Springer

Silvia Exenberger
Barbara Juen
Department of Psychology
University of Innsbruck
Innsbruck
Austria

ISSN 2211-7644   ISSN 2211-7652 (electronic)
ISBN 978-94-007-7518-3   ISBN 978-94-007-7519-0   (eBook)
DOI 10.1007/978-94-007-7519-0
Springer Dordrecht Heidelberg New York London

Library of Congress Control Number: 2013946951

Printed on acid-free paper

Springer is part of Springer Science+Business Media (www.springer.com)

Foreword

What constitutes a good life in childhood after a natural disaster? How do children view their well-being and how do they negotiate caregivers with restrictions and hope? Silvia Exenberger's and Barbara Juen's book on "Well-Being, Resilience and Quality of Life from Children's Perspectives: A Contextualized Approach" offers an innovative view on child well-being in the light of resources as well as in the light of the vulnerability in childhood. Its topic on children and caregivers in the post-Tsunami regions and their concepts of what constitutes a good life for children is an important issue in the general field of child well-being.

At the beginning, the Authors explore the broad view on child well-being and the quality of life research. As a result, the contributions to the first part of the book represent the entire spectrum of topics in the international discussion: the first concern is the conceptual issues, the second is the measurement of differences within one heterogeneous nation by looking at, for example, childhood in rural regions and comparing it to a childhood in metropolitan areas, the third is international comparisons, the fourth is the influence of data-based research on policymaking, the fifth is the fundamental question regarding which domains exert the greatest influence on child well-being in order to draw conclusions on where policy should intervene, and finally the sixth is the need to ask the children themselves.

I would like to take a closer look at the question how the well-being of children relates to that of families, how the concept of vulnerability could be seen, and what role do the children themselves play in this process.

Relations within the family and parental care are often applied as indicators of child well-being and they seem to play an important role. However, I would like to focus attention on something else: on the relation of child well-being to family well-being. Or, to put it differently: How does child policy relate to family policy? Even a superficial international comparison reveals how child and family well-being overlap: they overlap in access to gainful employment, in the quality of care facilities, in the normative ideas on a "good childhood and family," and in the work-life balance. But now this study shows more than that: It took a closer look at the long-term effects of trauma in children aged 7–15 and it realized a culture-sensitive and generational-sensitive approach. The researchers experienced the interdependence of the Indian culture where the study was located and that gave the first impression on children's and caregivers' roots of thinking about well-being: "However, with regard to the research it became very clear in order to understand well-being in the given sub-culture children and caregivers need to be consulted." (p. 3).

I would like to figure out another topic: the topic of resilience and vulnerability. In this book, the Authors focus on resilience and differentiated between two waves of research on resilience. With respect to a socio-ecological definition Exenberger and Juen follow Michael Ungar's definition of resilience and define resilience as the capacity of individuals to navigate their way to resources that sustain their well-being and their capacity individually and collectively to negotiate for these resources. This perspective offers a child-sensitive approach as resilience cannot be gained explicitly through internal resources, but also external ones are needed.

In this field of research on resilience and vulnerability we can find a diagnosis of the parental need for security as well: children are considered to be at risk, and they are particularly insecure in public spaces. This is reflected in the fact that protection is one of the fundamental orientations of the UN Convention on the Rights of the Child alongside development, education, and participation. Not only parents and other adults in their concrete interaction with children but also institutions in their formal shaping of childhood develop and establish more or less successful strategies to make the childhood life phase as secure and safe from harm as possible. However, what exactly is perceived as a threat or a risk depends decisively on the contexts in which children are growing up: often mentioned is the educational level and status of their parents, the public discourses over risks, or the norms of the state and civil society. In addition, it is precisely social contexts that are linked closely to normative attributions.

But this book decisively makes clear how a disaster like the Tsunami in 2004, confronts us with completely other questions on resilience, well-being, and vulnerability. It makes clear that these concepts only can be understood considering the social and ecological context of the concerned children and caregivers.

Finally, we have to discuss with respect to this excellent study whether research can and should fulfill the function of helping to represent the interests of children on the basis of data, particularly when based on quantitative and qualitative surveys of children as the experts on themselves. The orientation toward children's rights of access to all areas of society plays a strong role in the development of the child well-being approach. One element is asking the children themselves, and even younger children.

We need more case-studies in this sense of context-sensitivity and a strong interest in children's concepts on well-being in such circumstances like in the post-Tsunami regions.

Sabine Andresen

Preface

The Imperative Necessity to Give People a Voice

The project 'Three years post-Tsunami: Long-term effects of trauma in children aged 7–15—A culture-sensitive approach' received funding from the European Community's Seventh Framework Programme, Marie Curie Actions, International Outgoing Fellowships. The first Author was awarded with that funding, holding a post-doctoral position. The second Author, together with an Indian cooperation partner—Prof. Kasi Sekar from the Department of Psychiatric Social Work, National Institute of Mental Health and Neurosciences (NIMHANS)—a deemed university based in Bangalore—was supervising the entire research process throughout the project duration. The cultural adequacy of the research process was guaranteed through this cooperation as all steps during the research were discussed in face-to-face meetings. Moreover, in December 2008, the first Author received a training at NIMHANS on 'Psychosocial Care for Disaster Management' by the Indian cooperation partner. The second cooperation partner in India was SOS Children's Villages India. Their support was crucial and indispensable as they helped with the recruitment of child and adult participants and established some other necessary cooperation.

The duration of the whole project was from October 2008 to October 2011. Data collection and partly data processing took place in Tamil Nadu and UT Puducherry, South India, where the first Author lived with her family from October 2008 to September 2010. The present research was originally planned as one—not too large—segment of the entire project, but quickly became more and more important once the first Author tried to settle down in India. Already in the first days, the main features of collectivism (interdependence, norms as determinants for social behavior, etc.—see Triandis 1995) could be experienced first-hand. For example, it was not possible to open a bank account without any reference letter of just any person who was already a customer. Consequently, there was no alternative but to talk to Indians and to ask for their help. Once the first step toward inter-dependence and social networking was accomplished, we were part of the huge 'Indian family' and at the same time still considered as outsiders and strangers. But, this is another feature of Indian culture—unification of inconsistencies without causing any dissonance (Sinha et al. 2001). However, with regard to the research, it became very clear in order to understand well-being in the given subculture children and caregivers need to be consulted.

The book starts with a focus on the origin of the social indicator movement and gives a review of the literature on the concepts of quality of life, (subjective) well-being, and resilience. Delineations of the three concepts and their interplay, especially their intersection, are assumed to capture a full understanding of child well-being. In the subsequent chapter, the force of culture on child development will be highlighted. Based on the literature, it will be shown how two prototypical environments (rural subsistence-based and urban Western environment) favor either the independent or interdependent self-model, which in turn have implications on what competencies are valued in a specific culture and what determines subjective well-being. Consequently, our understanding of child well-being will be fully viewed against the background of culture. The Chap. 2 deals with shifts and changes within in the child well-being indicator movement and highlights important trends of child well-being measurements. The literature review of this book closes with a comparison of domains and indicators of current evidence-based national composite child well-being indices and child well-being indices from children's points of view.

In the subsequent chapters, the own research on the development of child well-being indicators 4 years after the Indian Ocean Tsunami disaster will be presented. The first part of the study gives Tsunami-affected children and their caregivers a voice to formulate in their words what constitutes child well-being for them in the given circumstances. The child well-being concepts of caregivers and those of children will be processed in detail and contrasted. In a new chapter, the second part of the study—the introduction of a child well-being index out of the developed indicators—is described. This index became part of a questionnaire battery that aimed to capture children's and mothers' own (mental) health status and resources. In this questioning, which was part of the larger project, a third group of children and their mothers were involved. All mothers gave answers in regard to their children's well-being. The strengths and shortcomings of this child well-being index are briefly discussed.

The book closes with four main conclusions that are reflected in a theoretical model toward contextualized child well-being indicators derived from the present research results.

References

Sinha, J. B. P., Sinha, T. N., Verma, J., & Sinha, R. B. N. (2001). Collectivism coexisting with individualism: An Indian scenario. *Asian Journal of Social Psychology, 4,* 133–145.
Triandis, H. C. (1995). *Individualism and collectivism.* Boulder: Westview Press.

Contents

Chapter 1
Social Indicators and the Concepts of Quality of Life, Subjective Well-Being, and Resilience

A Brief History of Social Indicators

The American Academy of Arts and Sciences (1962) got the assignment of the National Aeronautics and Space Administration (NASA) to investigate potential intended and unintended consequences of space exploration on the American society (American Academy of Arts and Sciences). Several scholars were involved in this multi-year project. They quickly discovered a lack of available data that measure and evaluate secondary effects of technology on people (Land 1983). It was then Raymond Bauer who filled this gap with the invention of the term and basic concept of 'social indicators' in 1966. His correspondent publication was considered as the project's most important. Even though the concern of societies with 'How we are doing?' and the usage of statistical indicators in order to measure social trends already existed for a long time, Bauer's publication launched the so called 'social indicators movement' (Noll 2002). He defined social indicators as

> ... statistics, statistical series, and all other forms of evidence that enable us to assess where we stand and are going with respect to our values and goals, and to evaluate specific programs and determine their impact (Bauer 1966a, b, p. 1).

With the social indicators, a way was paved for evaluating and monitoring the condition of groups in a society over time (Land 2000). However, Bauer's book was not an isolated event. In the same year of its appearance, President Johnson placed an order with the Secretary of Health, Education and Welfare—Wilbur J. Cohen:

> ... to develop the necessary social statistics and indicators to supplement those prepared by the Bureau of Labor Statistics and the Council of Economic Advisers (USDHEW 1969, p. 3).

In the introduction of the resulting publication *Toward a Social Report* (*TSR*), the shortcomings of the economic indicators became very clear. There was an explicit need of social indicators with the purpose of getting an idea how well-off people are. The development of a comprehensive set of social indicators presented

S. Exenberger and B. Juen, *Well-Being, Resilience and Quality of Life*
from Children's Perspectives, SpringerBriefs in Well-Being and Quality of Life Research,
DOI: 10.1007/978-94-007-7519-0_1, © The Author(s) 2014

in the TSR helped to find answers to the paradox of rising national income accompanied by lacking national well-being. The following six dimensions as basis of a regular system of social reporting were identified: health and illness; social mobility; physical environment; income and poverty; public order and safety; and learning, science, and art (USDHEW 1969). The definition of the term social indicator in the TSR emphasized a normative approach in judging real-life conditions. With this set of indicators, an instrument for improving public policy making was found in two ways: (1) visualization of social problems and (2) better evaluation of public programs' accomplishments (USDHEW 1969). Even though the TSR provided an important basis toward a social report, the authors were aware of its deficits. Information was not only needed on objective conditions, but also on how different groups of Americans perceived these living conditions (USDHEW 1969).

A few years later, in 1976, a new approach was developed to provide the missing information. Andrews and Withey (1976) published their book *Social Indicators of Well-Being: Americans' Perceptions of Life Quality*. More than 5000 American adults were interviewed about their perceptions of different life domains such as local government, home, family, and so on. Similarly, in the publication of Campbell et al. (1976) *The Quality of American Life: Perceptions, Evaluations and Satisfactions,* a quantitative analysis on subjective social indicators was introduced. Thus, with the quality of life concept and its objective and subjective social indicators as scientific measurements, a complement to the concept of material prosperity was developed (Noll 2002).

A Full Understanding of Child Well-Being

Different concepts are in use for the description of how well people are. Sometimes, terms such as well-being and quality of life are used interchangeably; at other times, they illustrate specific meanings (Veenhoven 2000). According to Veenhoven (2000) all these terms, which stand for 'all that is good' like well-being, quality of life, and happiness, signify evaluations. However, for the purpose of the present book, the concepts of (a) quality of life (briefly defined as objective well-being and subjective domain satisfaction), (b) (subjective) well-being (briefly defined as subjective life satisfaction and frequent joy), and (c) resilience (briefly defined as ability to navigate through adversities toward well-being) will be delineated (see below for full definitions of these three concepts). Through the attempt to define these concepts, it soon becomes clear that not the delineation of these concepts make up a full understanding of child well-being, but their interplay and where they overlap. Consequently, the intersection of these three concepts needs to be reflected in order to capture a full understanding of children's well-being, especially when they live and grow up in adverse situations (see Fig. 1.1).

Fig. 1.1 A full
understanding of child well-
being: An intersection of the
three concepts of quality of
life, well-being, and
resilience

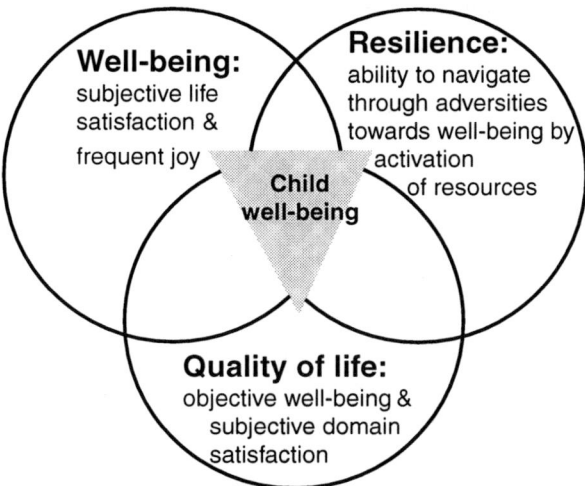

Quality of Life

With the invention of social indicators in the 1960s, instruments to measure quality of life and its changes over time were found (Casas 2011; Land et al. 2007). Cummins (1996, 1997) described two basic approaches to the definition and measurement of the quality-of-life construct: (1) a single unitary entity ('How do you feel about your life as a whole?') and (2) a composition of distinct life domains. Cummins (1997) viewed the limitations of the former approach. On the one hand, it cannot be applied to measurements on the objective axis, and on the other hand, only a rough estimation of perceived well-being is resulting. Concerning the latter approach, the possible number of life domains is large. Consequently, Cummins (1997) reduced this quantity by reviewing 27 definitions of life quality that attempted to identify discrete domains. Out of this review, he concluded that the following seven domains are intended to cover the spectrum of life quality:

- emotion (emotional well-being—in some form satisfaction, happiness, self-esteem etc.)
- health
- intimacy (social and family connections)
- material (material wealth or well-being)
- productivity (work or other form of productive activity)
- safety
- community.

According to Cummins

it is an imperative that all definitions and models of life quality be referenced to the general population both in their conception and in their operational measurement (Cummins 1997, p.127).

Another conclusion that Cummins drew out of his review was that quality of life refers to two axes: an objective and a subjective one.

Objective and Subjective Quality of Life

The history of the social indicators movement—as briefly described above—holds two conceptual approaches to the quality-of-life construct. The publications of Bauer and the USDHEW emphasized the objective components of life quality. These are based on observable and quantifiable facts related to various objective criteria for 'good' life such as number of friends, poverty rate, and unemployment rate (Cummins 2005; Diener and Suh 1997; Huebner et al. 2012). The so-called objective axis reflects culturally normative values of well-being and people's actual circumstances of living (Cummins 1997). In contrast to the objective social indicators, the publications of Andrews and Withey (1976) as well as Campbell et al. (1976) were targeted on subjective measurements. This approach relies on the individual's own judgment and evaluation about his/her social life conditions (e.g., job satisfaction). The quality of life is defined in terms of individuals' experiences (Noll 2002). According to Cummins (2005), to encompass the totality of human life, both objective and subjective dimensions must be included in the quality-of-life construct. Moreover, the correlation between the objective and subjective components is normally weak (Cummins 2000). The separateness of these two dimensions was already indicated in the TSR (USDHEW 1969) as an increase in population wealth did not implicate an improved experience of living. Subjective quality of life (respectively, subjective well-being according to Diener and Suh (1997)) is remarkably stable across time (Cummins et al. 2012; Eid and Diener 2004; Heady and Wearing 1989). In 1998, Cummins introduced the term 'homeostasis' to describe the basic mechanism underpinning subjective well-being (SWB) management (Cummins 2010; Cummins et al. 2012). According to Cummins (2010), homeostatical systems actively maintain SWB around its set point through external (e.g., money) and internal (e.g., automatic processes of adaptation) buffers. However, if a major life event (e.g., death of own child) constitutes an insurmountable challenge to SWB, then homeostasis fails (Cummins 2000, for a detailed review see Cummins et al. 2012).

To sum up, Diener and Suh (1997) pointed out the methodologically and conceptually complementary moments of the different approaches in order to measure the complexity and diversity of the quality-of-life construct. In their opinion, to understand human quality of life, objective and subjective social indicators as well as economic indices are needed (Diener and Suh 1997; Diener et al. 2003).

Defining Social Indicators and Quality of Life

Before turning to the SWB research, some terms need to be defined as they are used differently in the literature. These terms will be understood and used throughout this book according to the following definitions.

> The term *social indicator* is used to denote a statistic that is supposed to have some significance for measuring the quality of life (Sirgy et al. 2006, p. 344).

Objective and Subjective Indicators

Some researchers use the term 'social indicator' (e.g., Diener and Suh 1997) as a synonym for 'objective indicator' in terms of Sirgy et al. (2006), but here, the definition by Sirgy et al. (2006) for objective and subjective indicators is as follows:

> Social indicators that refer to personal feelings, attitudes, preferences, opinions, judgments or beliefs of some sort are called *subjective indicators*, e.g., satisfaction with one's health, attitudes towards science or scientists, beliefs about the danger of some new technology. Social indicators that refer to things that are relatively easily observable and measurable are called *objective indicators*, e.g., the height and weight of people, numbers of automobiles manufactured or sold each year, numbers of people employed in research and development (Sirgy et al. 2006, pp. 344–345).

Quality of Life

There is a lack of consensus on the definition of the 'quality of life' concept (Taillefer et al. 2003; Veenhoven 2000; Ventegodt et al. 2011). It is used in different disciplines (e.g., philosophy, medicine, economics, psychology, etc.) and defined differently across these disciplines (Eckermann 2012). According to Eckermann (2012), there are two common features across the variety of definitions. First is the adoption of a positive foundation about the 'good life'; second, the integration of both indicators (subjective and objective) in the quality-of-life construct. Quality of life is both objective and subjective; consequently, a comprehensive definition comprises both dimensions (Cummins 1997, 2000, 2005):

> … Objective domains comprise culturally-relevant measures of objective well-being. Subjective domains comprise domain satisfaction weighted by their importance to the individual (Cummins 1997, p. 6).

Well-Being and Subjective Well-Being

The subjective approach to the 'quality-of-life definition' is most associated with the subjective well-being tradition (Diener and Suh 1997; Sirgy et al. 2006) where people's evaluation of their lives constitutes an indispensable component of positive psychological health (Diener et al. 1998). To fully conceive subjective well-being, the origin of the well-being concept, which is embedded in a historical and philosophical context, must be considered. Its trail can be traced back to the ancient Greece (Diener 1984; Haybron 2008). Even though current research shows that well-being originates from five major philosophical theories (Hayborn 2008), the two most prominent approaches according to Ryan and Deci (2001), Joshanloo (2013)—hedonism and eudaimonism—will be described here.

The Hedonic and Eudaimonic View on Well-Being

The theory of *hedonism* is derived from the Greek philosopher Aristippus from the fourth century B.C. This theory taught that the experience of pleasure is the highest good and proper aim in human life. And happiness is the totality of one's hedonic moments. Hedonism as a view on well-being has a broad focus and consists of subjective happiness and concerns the experience of pleasure (Ryan and Deci 2001). Hedonism is supposed to focus on positive feelings per se (King 2008) and the hedonic quality of individuals' experiences matters ultimately for their well-being (Haybron 2008).

The counterpart to the hedonistic approach of well-being constitutes the eudaimonic one. Etymologically, *eudaimonia* consists of the Greek 'eu' (good) and 'daimon' (spirit). Within the term is a notion of fortune, for having a good 'daimon', a guiding spirit, on your side (McMahon 2008). Eudaimonia is a central concept of Aristotle described as the

> ... highest of all human goods as the realization of one's true potential (Ryff and Singer 1998, p. 2).

From a eudaimonic view, the criterion for happiness is not the actor's subjective judgment. A desirable state is judged from a value framework (Diener 1984). Within the eudaimonic account Ryff et al. (2004) identified six key dimensions of well-being or positive health: autonomy, environmental mastery, personal growth, positive relations with others, purpose in life, and self-acceptance. This rather objectivist view on well-being and health challenged the SWB models of well-being. Even though Diener et al. (1998) valued Ryff and Singer's (1998) emphasis on positive health, they viewed the absence of SWB in their formulation of health and the good life as a 'conspicuous omission' (p. 33). Diener et al. (1998) argued that SWB allows people to tell researchers what makes their life good, instead of letting experts define well-being for them.

The controversy about the two approaches of well-being, which had its origin in ancient days, is not yet resolved. Even though empirical research of hedonic psychology often falls under the realm of SWB, which has a hedonic component (Larsen and Eid 2008), SWB is more than pure hedonism. People not only want to feel happy, but also want to feel positive about what they are achieving that they believe is valuable and worthwhile (Diener and Tov 2012). Consequently, modern conceptions of well-being stress a multi-dimensional view that includes both the hedonic as well as eudaimonic aspect (Diener and Tov 2012; Ryan and Deci 2001).

Subjective Well-Being

In general, SWB is a person's evaluation about his or her life. Diener (1984) distinguished three components of subjective well-being: life satisfaction, positive affect, and negative affect. Life satisfaction comprises a person's evaluation about his or her life as a whole (Diener 2006). In 1999, Diener et al. extended the definition of SWB with people's satisfaction in specific life domains such as satisfaction with health, social relations, etc. Researchers often differentiate between two broad components of SWB: the affective and the cognitive one. The latter is represented in terms of conscious thought and judging whether life is satisfying and fulfilling or not (Diener and Tov 2012). In contrast, moods and emotions constitute immediate evaluations of events that occur in people's lives and reflect the amount of pleasant and unpleasant feelings about these experiences (Schimmack 2008). The independence of positive and negative affect was uncovered by Bradburn in 1969, when he published his classic book *The Structure of Psychological Well-Being* (Diener 1984). High levels of positive affect are expressed by high energy and pleasurable engagement, whereas sadness and lethargy characterize low positive affect levels. In contrast, negative affect includes unpleasant moods and emotions. A variety of aversive mood states such as anger, fear, guilt, etc. is subsumed. Low negative affect is expressed by a state of calmness and serenity (Diener 2006; Watson et al. 1988).

Defining Well-Being, Subjective Well-Being, and Happiness

As already indicated above, no single concept represents the full nature of well-being. There are various types of well-being which correlate only moderately with each other (Diener and Tov 2012).

Well-Being

Recently, Diener and his colleagues developed a temporal model of well-being in a table format that illustrates the multi-faceted phenomenon of well-being and the requirement for multi-pronged assessment (Diener and Tov 2012). The model comprises a temporal sequence starting at external events and circumstances and moving through experiences to recall and global evaluations. Pleasant and unpleasant emotions as well as cognitive judgments (global and domain specific) can be assessed at different stages of the temporal sequence. The authors also included motivational and other concepts of well-being such as optimism and trust (Diener and Tov 2012).

According to Diener and Tov, each of these different facets can be relevant to the quality of life.

Subjective Well-Being, and Happiness

SWB is known by lay people as 'happiness' or 'satisfaction' (Diener et al. 2003). Diener et al. (1997) define SWB as judging life positively and feeling good:

> Thus a person is said to have high [subjective well-being] if she or he experiences life satisfaction and frequent joy, and only infrequently experiences unpleasant emotions such as sadness and anger. Contrariwise, a person is said to have low [subjective well-being] if she or he is dissatisfied with life, experiences little joy and affection and frequently feels negative emotions such as anger or anxiety (Diener et al. 1997, p. 25).

The definition of happiness according to Veenhoven (2008) is close to Diener et al.'s definition of SWB. Also Veenhoven differentiates between cognitive and affective appraisals of life, but he does not view life satisfaction as a mere cognitive evaluation like Diener. An overall judgment of life draws on *cognitive comparison* with standards of the good life and *affective information* from how one feels (Veenhoven 2008).

In this book, we follow Veenhoven's language and use 'overall happiness' synonymously with SWB (Veenhoven 2008).

Resilience

The term resilience (Latin *resilire* 'to recoil', from *re-* 'back' and *salire* 'to jump') (The New Oxford Dictionary of English 1998) is described within the materials sciences as

> ... the ability of a material to resume its original shape or position after being spent, stretched or compressed (Goldstein and Brooks 2006, p. 8).

The etymology of the term resilience and its usage in material sciences reflect the image of resilience in the psychological sciences as the ability of individuals to recover from serious threats. Masten (2001) defines resilience as

> ...a class of phenomena characterized by good outcomes in spite of serious threats to adaptation or development (Masten 2001, p. 228).

Masten's definition implies two major judgments for the identification of resilience. Firstly, the individual was exposed to adversity, and secondly, the quality of adaptation was positively evaluated. In this sense, resilience is in contrast to the concepts of competence and well-being (Masten 2001; Masten and Coatsworth 1998).

This individually focused view of resilience terms Ungar (2012) 'the first interpretation of resilience' (p. 13). Even though different authors speak about four waves within the resilience research (e.g., Sapienza and Masten 2011), the two broadest approaches according to Ungar (2012) will be mentioned here.

First Wave of Resilience Research: Individual Capacity

One of the most striking results of Werner's and Smith's longitudinal pioneer study on resilience with an entire birth cohort born in 1955 on the Hawaiian island of Kauai showed that one-third of the children who had faced multiple risks grew into competent adults (Werner and Smith 1992; Werner 1993). Their findings shifted the primary assumption of scholars and mass media in the 1970s that resilient children are invulnerable (Masten 2001; Werner and Smith 1992). Over the years, resilience research proved the ordinariness of the phenomena, showing that there is nothing 'remarkable' or 'special' about resilient children, but a common operation of human adaptive systems (e.g., secure attachment) (Masten 2001). Within this so-called first wave of resilience research, specific attention was paid on the individual. The focus laid on the risk and protective factors, which were associated with an individual's ability to cope with challenging circumstances (Wright and Masten 2006). This initial research mainly identified personal competences that resilient individuals demonstrated in order to overcome adversities they experienced (Benard 2004).

The International Resilience Project went beyond this research focus and asked a new question what parents, teachers, other adults, and children themselves do to promote resilience in children (Grotberg 1997). The common thrust was that the universal capacity for resilience is developed and nurtured by the following factors: (1) *provided* around the child (e.g., access to health, education, and welfare; trusting relationships), (2) *acquired* by the child (e.g., impulse control; intellectual skills), and (3) *developed* within the child (e.g., a sense of being lovable; autonomy) (Grotberg 1998). Grotberg (1997, 1998) labeled the different sources of resilience as I HAVE (external resources), I CAN (interpersonal skills), and I AM (inner strengths).

The results of the International Resilience Project already point out the importance of the availability of external resources for an individual in order to be resilient. As a consequence, resilience goes more and more beyond the dominance of a Westernized conceptualization as an intra-psychic construct—one of Ungar's (2007) major critique on the first wave or resilience research—toward a contextualized approach (Ungar 2012).

Second Wave of Resilience Research: A Social Ecological Approach

In the second wave of resilience research, larger contextual concerns were addressed. Resilience was embedded in developmental and ecological systems, and research focused on the understanding of the complex and systemic interactions that shaped both negative and positive developmental outcomes (Wright and Masten 2006). Ungar (2012) assumes that environments perhaps even count more than individual capacity as antecedents of positive coping after an individual's exposure to adversity. His assumption broadens the view on resilience as health is no longer understood as an individual experience. Emphasis is put on the

> … adequate provision of health resources necessary to achieve good outcomes in spite of serious threats to adaptation or development (Ungar 2005, p. 429).

This understanding of resilience highlights the social context and views resilience as dependent on access to resources (Ungar 2005). According to Ungar (2011), the study of resilience should first focus on the context and then on the child. On that note, a child can only be as much resilient as the surrounding environment or system gives him or her the chance (Afifi and MacMillan 2011).

Defining Resilience

In this book, a social ecological definition of resilience is applied:

> In the context of exposure to significant adversity, resilience is both the capacity of individuals to navigate their way to the psychological, social, cultural, and physical resources that sustain their well-being, and their capacity individually and collectively to negotiate for these resources to be provided and experienced in culturally meaningful ways (Ungar 2008, p. 225).

The first concept of *navigation* implies personal agency and puts the focus on the individual. The second concept of *negotiation* attributes meaning to the resources that are available and are defined as health-enhancing in a given culture (Ungar 2011).

References

Afifi, T. O., & MacMillan, H. L. (2011). Resilience following child maltreatment: A review of protective factors. *Canadian Journal of Psychiatry—Revue Canadienne de Psychiatrie, 56*(5), 266–272.

American Academy of Arts and Sciences. (1962). Space exploration and society. http://www.amacad.org/projects%5C1960s_sci.aspx. Accessed 9 June 2013.

Andrews, F. M., & Withey, S. B. (1976). *Social indicators of well-being: Americans' Perceptions of life quality*. New York: Plenum.

Bauer, R. (1966a). Detection and anticipation of impact: The nature of the task. In R. A. Bauer (Ed.), *Social indicators* (pp. 1–67). Cambridge: M.I.T. Press.

Bauer, R. A. (Ed.). (1966b). *Social indicators*. Cambridge: M.I.T. Press.

Benard, B. (2004). *Resiliency: What we have learned*. San Francisco: WestEd.

Campbell, A., Converse, P. E., & Rodgers, W. L. (1976). *The quality of American life: perceptions, evaluations and satisfactions*. New York: Russell Sage Foundation.

Casas, F. (2011). Subjective social indicators and child and adolescent well-being. *Child Indicators Research, 4*(4), 555–575.

Cummins, R. A. (1996). The domains of life satisfaction: An attempt to order chaos. *Social Indicators Research, 38*, 303–328.

Cummins, R. A. (1997). Assessing quality of life. In R. I. Brown (Ed.), *Quality of life for people with disabilities* (2nd ed., pp. 116–150). Cheltenham: Stanley Thornes.

Cummins, R. A. (2000). Objective and subjective quality of life: An interactive model. *Social Indicators Research, 52*, 55–72.

Cummins, R. A. (2005). Moving from the quality of life concept to a theory. *Journal of Intellectual Disability Research, 49*(10), 699–706.

Cummins, R. A. (2010). Subjective well-being, homeostatically protected mood and depression: A synthesis. *Journal of Happiness Studies, 11*, 1–17.

Cummins, R. A., Lau, A. L. D., & Davern, M. T. (2012). Subjective wellbeing homeostasis. In K. C. Land, A. C. Michalos, & M. J. Sirgy (Eds.), *Handbook of social indicators and quality of life research* (pp. 79–98). New York: Springer.

Diener, E. (1984). Subjective well-being. *Psychological Bulletin, 95*(3), 542–575.

Diener, E. (2006). Guidelines for national indicators of subjective well-being and ill-being. *Applied Research in Quality of Life, 1*, 151–157.

Diener, E., & Suh, E. (1997). Measuring quality of life: Economic, social, and subjective indicators. *Social Indicators Research, 40*, 189–216.

Diener, E., & Tov, W. (2012). National accounts of well-being. In K. C. Land, A. C. Michalos, & M. J. Sirgy (Eds.), *Handbook of social indicators an quality of life research* (pp. 137–157). New York: Springer.

Diener, E., Oishi, S., & Lucas, R. E. (2003). Personality, culture, and subjective well-being: Emotional and cognitive evaluations of life. *Annual Review of Psychology, 54*, 403–425.

Diener, E., Sapyta, J. J., & Suh, E. (1998). Subjective well-being is essential to well-being. *Psychological Inquiry, 9*(1), 33–37.

Diener, E., Suh, E., & Oishi, S. (1997). Recent findings on subjective well-being. *Indian Journal of Clinical Psychology, 24*(1), 25–41.

Eckermann, E. (2012). The quality of life of adults. In K. C. Land, A. C. Michalos, & M. J. Sirgy (Eds.), *Handbook of social indicators and quality of life research* (pp. 373–380). New York: Springer.

Eid, M., & Diener, E. (2004). Global judgements of subjective well-being: Situational variability and long-term stability. *Social Indicators Research, 65*, 245–277.

Goldstein, S., & Brooks, R. B. (2006). Why study resilience? In S. Goldstein & R. B. Brooks (Eds.), *Handbook of resilience in children* (pp. 3–15). New York: Springer Science+Business Media, Inc.

Grotberg, E. H. (1997). The International Resilience Project: Findings from the research and effectiveness of interventions. http://resilnet.uiuc.edu/library/grotb97a.html. Accessed 9 June 2013.

Grotberg, E. H. (1998). The International Resilience Project. http://resilnet.uiuc.edu/library/grotb98a.html. Accessed 9 June 2013.

Haybron, D. M. (2008). Philosophy and the science of subjective well-being. In M. Eid & R. J. Larsen (Eds.), *The science of subjective well-being* (pp. 17–43). New York: The Guilford Press.

Headey, B., & Wearing, A. (1989). Personality, life events, and subjective well-being: Toward a dynamic equilibrium model. *Journal of Personality and Social Psychology, 57*(4), 731–739.

Huebner, E. S., Gilman, R., & Ma, C. (2012). Perceived quality of life of children and youth. In K. C. Land, A. C. Michalos, & M. J. Sirgy (Eds.), *Handbook of social indicators and quality of life research* (pp. 355–372). New York: Springer.

Joshanloo, M. (2013). Eastern conceptualizations of happiness: Fundamental differences with Western views. *Journal of Happiness Studies,* doi:10.1007/s10902-013-9431-1.

King, L. A. (2008). Interventions for enhancing subjective well-being: Can we make people happier and should we? In M. Eid & R. J. Larsen (Eds.), *The science of subjective well-being* (pp. 431–448). New York: The Guilford Press.

Land, K. C. (1983). Social indicators. *Annual Review of Sociology, 9,* 1–26.

Land, K. C. (2000). Social indicators. In E. F. Borgatta & R. J. V. Montgomery (Eds.), *Encyclopedia of sociology* (2nd ed., Vol. 4, pp. 2682–2690). New York: Macmillan Reference USA.

Land, K. C., Lamb, V. L., Meadows, S. O., & Taylor, A. (2007). Measuring trends in child well-being: An evidence-based approach. *Social Indicators Research, 80,* 105–132.

Larsen, R. J., & Eid, M. (2008). Ed Diener and the science of subjective well-being. In M. Eid & R. J. Larsen (Eds.), *The science of subjective well-being* (pp. 1–13). New York: The Guilford Press.

Masten, A. S. (2001). Ordinary magic. *American Psychologist, 56*(3), 227–238.

Masten, A. S., & Coatsworth, J. D. (1998). The development of competence in favorable and unfavorable environments. *American Psychologist, 53*(2), 205–220.

McMahon, D. M. (2008). The pursuit of happiness in history. In M. Eid & R. J. Larsen (Eds.), *The science of subjective well-being* (pp. 80–93). New York: The Guilford Press.

Noll, H–. H. (2002). Social indicators and quality of life research: Background, achievements and current trends. In N. Genov (Ed.), *Advances in sociological knowledge over half a century* (pp. 168–206). Paris: International Social Science Council.

Resilience. (1998). *The new Oxford Dictionary of English* (p. 1579). Oxford: Oxford University Press.

Ryan, R. M., & Deci, E. L. (2001). On happiness and human potentials: A review of research on hedonic and eudaimonic well-being. *Annual Review of Psychology, 52,* 141–166.

Ryff, C. D., & Singer, B. (1998). The contours of positive human health. *Psychological Inquiry, 9*(1), 1–28.

Ryff, C. D., Singer, B. H., & Dienberg Love, G. (2004). Positive health: Connecting well-being with biology. *Philosophical Transactions of the Royal Society of London, 359,* 1383–1394. doi:10.1098/rstb.2004.1521.

Sapienza, J. K., & Masten, A. S. (2011). Understanding and promoting resilience in children and youth. *Current Opinion in Psychiatry, 24*(4), 267–273.

Schimmack, U. (2008). The structure of subjective well-being. In M. Eid & R. J. Larsen (Eds.), *The science of subjective well-being* (pp. 97–123). New York: The Guilford Press.

Sirgy, M. J., Michalos, A. C., Ferriss, A. L., Easterlin, R. A., Patrick, D., & Pavot, W. (2006). The quality of life (QOL) research movement: Past, present, and future. *Social Indicators Research, 76,* 343–466.

Taillefer, M.-C., Dupuis, G., Roberge, M.-A., & Le May, S. (2003). Health-related quality of life models: Systematic review of the literature. *Social Indicators Research, 64,* 293–323.

Ungar, M. (2005). Pathways to resilience among children in child welfare, corrections, mental health and educational settings: Navigation and Negotiation. *Child and Youth Care Forum, 34*(6), 423–444.

Ungar, M. (2008). Resilience across cultures. *British Journal of Social Work, 38*, 218–235.

Ungar, M. (2011). The social ecology of resilience: Addressing contextual and cultural ambiguity of a nascent construct. *American Journal of Orthopsychiatry, 81*(1), 1–17.

Ungar, M. (2012). Social ecologies and their contribution to resilience. In M. Ungar (Ed.), *The social ecology of resilience* (pp. 13–31). New York: Springer.

Ungar, M., Brown, M., Liebenberg, L., Othman, R., Kwong, W. M., Armstrong, M., et al. (2007). Unique pathways to resilience across cultures. *Adolescence, 42*(166), 287–310.

U.S. Department of Health, Education, Welfare (USDHEW). (1969). Toward a social report. Washington D.C.: U.S. Government Printing Office.

Veenhoven, R. (2000). The four qualities of life. Ordering concepts and measures of the good life. *Journal of Happiness Studies, 1*, 1–39.

Veenhoven, R. (2008). Sociological theories of subjective well-being. In M. Eid & R. J. Larsen (Eds.), *The science of subjective well-being* (pp. 44–61). New York: The Guilford Press.

Ventegodt, S., Omar, H. A., & Merrick, J. (2011). Quality of life as medicine: Interventions that induce salutogenesis. A review of the literature. *Social Indicators Research, 100*, 415–433.

Watson, D., Lee, A. C., & Tellegen, A. (1988). Development and validation of brief measures of positive and negative affect: The PANAS scales. *Journal of Personality and Social Psychology, 54*(6), 1063–1070.

Werner, E. E. (1993). Risk, resilience, and recovery: Perspectives from the Kauai longitudinal study. *Development and Psychopathology, 5*, 503–515.

Werner, E. E., & Smith, R. S. (1992). *Overcoming the odds*. Ithaca: Cornell University Press.

Wright, M. O. D., & Masten, A. S. (2006). Resilience processes in development. In S. Goldstein & R. B. Brooks (Eds.), *Handbook of resilience in children* (pp. 17–37). New York: Springer Science+Busines Media, Inc.

Chapter 2
Culture and Child Well-Being

Culture constructs the way how human beings perceive the reality. It shapes perceptual and experiential patterns, which people use to describe, understand, predict, and control the world around them (Marsella 2010). According to Marsella (2010) and Marsella and Christopher (2004), culture can be defined as follows:

> Shared learned behavior and meanings acquired in life activity contexts that are passed on from generation to another for purposes of promoting survival, adaptation, and adjustment. These behaviors and meanings are dynamic, and are responsive to change and modification in response to individual, societal, and environmental demands and pressures. Culture is represented *externally* in artifacts, roles, settings, and institutions. Culture is represented *internally* in values, beliefs, expectations, consciousness, epistemology (i.e., ways of knowing), ontology, and praxiology, personhood, and world views. Cultures can be situational, temporary, or enduring. (Marsella 2010, p. 19)

Keller (2007) views this conceptualization of culture as a dynamic and socially interactive process. Within this concept, culture is represented inside and outside the individual. Shared meanings (cultural interpretation) constitute the 'inside', and the 'outside' is manifested in shared activities (cultural practices) (Greenfield et al. 2003; Keller 2007).

Culture and Development

In 1953, Havighurst published his book 'Human Development and Education'. With this publication, he introduced the concept of developmental tasks. The central idea of this concept is that development is a learning process, which extends over the whole life span. Developmental tasks originate from the source of (a) the pressure of cultural processes upon the individual (e.g., participation as a socially responsible citizen of society), (b) physical maturation (e.g., learning to walk), and (c) an individual's personal values and aspirations (e.g., choosing and preparing for an occupation). Mainly, developmental tasks arise from combinations of these three factors acting together. Thus, at any stage in life, the individual is confronted with various developmental tasks that he or she has to accomplish

S. Exenberger and B. Juen, *Well-Being, Resilience and Quality of Life from Children's Perspectives*, SpringerBriefs in Well-Being and Quality of Life Research, DOI: 10.1007/978-94-007-7519-0_2, © The Author(s) 2014

(Havighurst 1953). According to Havighurst, the successful achievement leads to happiness and the success with later tasks, whereas failure leads to unhappiness, disapproval by the society, and presumable difficulty with future tasks. There are a series of universal developmental tasks that have evolved and have to be solved in culture-specific ways (Greenfield et al. 2003; Keller 2007). Developmental tasks (considering age and culture of a child) are also used as criteria to judge a child's developmental outcome after facing adversity (Masten et al. 1999). It emerges that cultural forces are crucial for the understanding of *what* is defined successful when completing a developmental task and *what* is viewed as a key competency in a given context. In terms of Ogbu's cultural–ecological theory (1981), competence is not universally defined but within the cultural and historical context in which children develop. Thus, the solution of the developmental tasks must be culturally sensitive so that locally defined competences are represented as positive adaptation in a given context (Keller 2007).

The value of various competencies is culturally dependent and rooted in cultural models of the self (Keller 2007). For example, 'conformity' of an individual can be viewed from different perspectives. On the one hand, it may reflect an inability to resist social pressure. On the other hand, conformity can show a willingness to be responsive to others and subordinate one's desires in order to maintain the relationship (Markus and Kitayama 2003). Markus and Kitayama (1991, 2003) assumed that the perceptions what individuals have about their self–other relations lead to two broad modes of being. Especially, to what extent individuals view themselves as separate from others or connected with others. On the basis of separation or connectedness between the self and others, the authors distinguished an independent from an interdependent self-construal. The term 'self-construal' they defined.

> … as patterns of past behavior, as well as patterns for one's current and future behavior …
> (Markus and Kitayama 2003, p. 280).

The distinction between an independent and an interdependent self-construal represents general tendencies that emerge when the members of a culture are considered as a whole. For example, the American view of the self is most characteristic for white, middle-class individuals with a European ethnic background, and may be less applicable to individuals belonging to another ethnic group or social class (Markus and Kitayama 1991). The idea of an unitary 'Western mind' was also challenged by Harkness et al. (2000) when analyzing US and Dutch parents' cultural models of the child both belonging to two socioeconomically similar populations. The two groups of parents recognized the same kinds of behavior as relevant to the constructs dependence and independence, but they highly differed in their interpretations of and responses to such behaviors.

Evolution of the Two Self-Models

Following an eco-cultural approach, which was pioneered by the anthropologists Beatrice and John Whiting (Keller 2007), the structure of the physical environment like climate (Van de Vliert et al. 1999), population parameters such as population density (Triandis 1995), and the socioeconomic structure (Triandis 1995) forms the framework for socialization strategies. Socialization strategies consist of ideas and practices that directly influence child development (Keller 2007). From an eco-cultural perspective, it can be assumed that social structures, which favor various developmental pathways, are created by certain environmental and economic conditions (Greenfield et al. 2003). In the following, two prototypical environments, which lead to respective family interaction patterns and consequently are responsible for the generation of the two models of self, are described briefly.

The Independent Self-Construal

In Western industrial societies, which are characterized by large-scale population, the independent self-model is common. The economy is money based with individual income varieties, and people face many daily anonymous encounters (Keller and Otto 2009). Education levels are high, and lifestyle is based on choice, individual freedom, and personal achievement (Tamis-LeMonda 2008; Triandis 1995). Due to affluence, high level of education, and alternative sources of old-age support, parents do not depend on their children later on. Parents value children because they imply joy, fun, companionship, and love (Aycicegi-Dinn and Kagitcibasi 2010). Children are brought up to be independent, self-sufficient, and autonomous (Kagitcibasi 2005). Markus and Kitayama (1991) refer an independent self-construal to an individual who is autonomous, unique, separate, competitive, and self-reliant. This construal places emphasis on self-enhancement, self-expression, and self-maximization (Markus and Kitayama 1991) and corresponds to the concept of individualism on a cultural level and idiocentrism on an individual level (Triandis 1995; Triandis and Suh 2002). Within the individualistic concept, the individual is given preference to the group (Triandis 1995). In terms of Kagitcibasi (2005), the individualistic worldview is expressed through the separate self, which captures the two dimensions of autonomy and separation.

The Interdependent Self-Construal

The *interdependent self-model* is prevalent in rural agrarian societies (Kagitcibasi 2005). They are characterized through high population density with low levels of affluence and subsistence-based economy. Formal education is predominantly basic (Keller 2007). The self is viewed as interdependent with in-groups or collectives and changes depending on the in-group or collective the individual is with. Examples for in-groups are family, tribe, and nation (Triandis 2004). The value of children for parents is reflected in the dependence of the family not only on adult offspring for its livelihood, but also when the children are young and needed to help with household chores (Aycicegi-Dinn and Kagitcibasi 2010). Thus, the independence of a child is not valued as the child may leave the family in order to realize his or her own interests (Kagitcibasi 2005). Obedience and respect to elders are considered as the highest values in parenting in many collectivist-oriented communities (Tamis-LeMonda et al. 2008). The interdependent self-construal refers to an individual who strongly feels that he or she belongs to a social group. The opinions held by significant others about the individual determine and organize to a large extent the actor's behavior (Markus and Kitayama 1991). People are motivated to be conform with relevant others; they accept hierarchy and their own role within this group and try to keep up group harmony (Keller 2003). The interdependent self-construal is the corresponding concept to collectivism on a cultural level and allocentrism on an individual level (Triandis 1995; Triandis and Suh 2002). In collectivistic cultures, individual interests are subordinated to the interests of the group (Triandis 1995). The family model of interdependence is dominant in collectivistic cultures and is defined by the dimensions of relatedness and heteronomy according to Kagitcibasi (2005).

Keller (2003) emphasized that the two self-construals are not dichotomous and mutually exclusive, but occur in particular mixtures in an individual. Trends of increased globalization, immigration, and technology call for changes in parents' and children's value systems (Tamis-LeMonda et al. 2008) and lead to a third model of the self-autonomous–relational self (Kagitcibasi 1996; Aycicegi-Dinn and Kagitcibasi 2010). The autonomous–relational self emerges through the global shift from the family model of interdependence to the family model of independence with urbanization and economic development (Kagitcibasi 1996, Aycicegi-Dinn and Kagitcibasi 2010). In general, scholars move beyond the grand division of collectivism and individualism toward an emphasis of coexistence of individualistic and collectivistic tendencies within individuals, families, and cultures (Sinha and Kumar 2004; Tamis-LeMonda2008; Triandis 1995).

Culture and SWB

As outlined above, culture selects one self-model over another. The respective self-construal as self-schema shapes and directs an individual's behavior in such a way that cultural core concerns are reflected (Lu et al. 2001). Thus, the meaning of happiness or SWB is molded by culture (Lu and Gilmour 2004), largely dependent on culture, and consequently cross-culturally variable (Uchida et al. 2004). Even though, it is agreed upon across cultures that happiness is a desirable, positive inner state of mind (Suh and Koo 2008), some remarkable differences between the Chinese (Lu 2001) and American students' definitions of happiness emerged (Lu and Gilmour 2004). The Asian respondents emphasized a harmonious homeostasis within the individual as well as between the individual and his/her surroundings comparable to the ancient *Yin–Yang* theory (Lu 2001). According to the Yin–Yang theory, which discusses changes not one-dimensional but from one extreme to another extreme (Ji et al. 2001), a clear dialectical view of the happiness–unhappiness relationship contrasted the American accounts of happiness (Lu 2001). Ji et al. (2001) assume that the belief in change has implications for psychological well-being, so that unhappiness is viewed as a less undesirable state in East Asians compared to Westerners. The individual-oriented SWB approach of Euro-Americans stressed the importance of personal accountability and an explicit pursuit of personal happiness (Lu and Gilmour 2004).

In an earlier study, Lu et al. (2001) described two ways to achieve happiness determined by an independent and interdependent self-construal, respectively. In an individualistic society, the belief about social interactions is based on control (Lu et al. 2001), which means the state of happiness can be reached through personal achievement (Uchida et al. 2004). In contrast, in a collectivistic culture, the self in relationship with others determines SWB. The preservation of harmony within social relationships is a cause for social interaction that leads to happiness (Uchida et al. 2004). Belief systems reflect norms and expectations of cultures and are transmitted from parents to children (Keller 2003).

To sum up, the two constructs of individualism and collectivism are useful and powerful to explain general patterns of differences and similarities between cultures (Kim-Prieto and Eid 2004; Triandis 1995). Following an eco-cultural approach, prototypical environments (rural subsistence-based and urban Western environment) favor the independent and the interdependent self-model (Markus and Kitayama 1991), which correspond to individualism and collectivism, respectively. The independent self-model views the self *separate from others,* whereas the interdependent self-model views the self *connected with others.* These divergent views of the self have implications on what competencies are valued in a specific culture (Keller 2003) and what determines happiness or SWB (Lu et al. 2001; Uchida et al. 2004).

At this point, it becomes clear that the claim to a full understanding of child well-being only can be accomplished if child well-being—as outlined in Fig. 2.1—is understood from the perspective of culture (see Fig. 2.1).

Fig. 2.1 Child well-being:
embedding in the cultural
setting

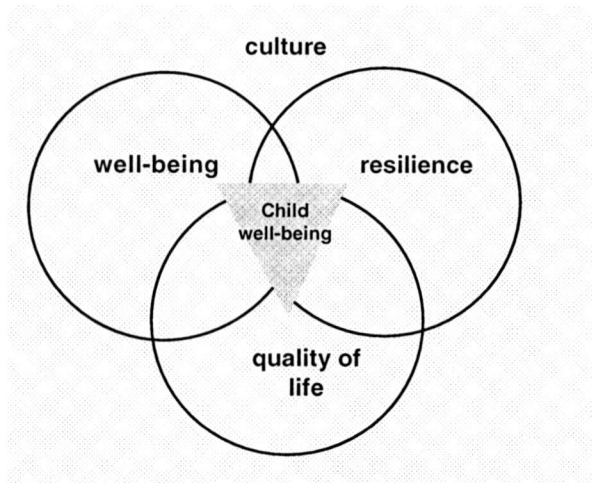

References

Aycicegi-Dinn, A., & Kagitcibasi, C. (2010). The value of children for parents in the minds of emerging adults. *Cross-Cultural Research, 44*(2), 174–205.

Greenfield, P. M., Keller, H., Fuligni, A., & Maynard, A. (2003). Cultural pathways through universal development. *Annual Review of Psychology, 54*, 461–490.

Harkness, S., Super, C. M., & Van Tijen, N. (2000). Individualism and the 'Western Mind' reconsidered: American and Dutch parents' ethnotheories of the child. In S. Harkness, C. Raeff, & C. M. Super (Eds.), *Variability of the social construction of the child* (pp. 23–39). San Francisco: Jossey Bass Publishers.

Havighurst, R. J. (1953). *Human development and education.* London: Longmans Green.

Ji, L.-J., Nisbett, R. E., & Su, Y. (2001). Culture, change, and prediction. *Psychological Science, 12*(6), 450–456.

Kagitcibasi, C. (1996). The autonomous-relational self: A new synthesis. *European Psychologist, 1*(3), 180–186.

Kagitcibasi, C. (2005). Autonomy and relatedness in cultural context. *Journal of Cross-Cultural Psychology, 36*(4), 403–422.

Keller, H. (2003). Socialization for competence: Cultural models of infancy. *Human Development, 46*, 288–311.

Keller, H. (2007). *Cultures of infancy.* New Jersey: Lawrence Erlbaum Associates.

Keller, H., & Otto, H. (2009). The cultural socialization of emotion regulation during infancy. *Journal of Cross-Cultural Psychology, 40*(6), 996–1011.

Kim-Prieto, C., & Eid, M. (2004). Norms for experiencing emotions in Sub-Saharan Africa. *Journal of Happiness Studies, 5*, 241–268.

Lu, L. (2001). Understanding happiness: A look into the Chinese folk psychology. *Journal of Happiness Studies, 2*, 407–432.

Lu, L., & Gilmour, R. (2004). Culture and concepts of happiness: Individual oriented and social oriented SWB. *Journal of Happiness Studies, 5*, 269–291.

Lu, L., Gilmour, R., Kao, S. F., Weng, T. H., Hu, C. H., Chern, J. G., et al. (2001). Two ways to achieve happiness: When the East meets the West. *Personality and Individual Differences, 30*, 1161–1174.

Markus, H. R., & Kitayama, S. (1991). Culture and the self: Implications for cognition, emotion and motivation. *Psychological Review, 98*(2), 224–253.

Markus, H. R., & Kitayama, S. (2003). Culture, self, and the reality of the social. *Psychological Inquiry, 14*(3&4), 277–283.

Marsella, A. J. (2010). Ethnocultural aspects of PTSD: An overview of concepts, issues, and treatments. *Traumatology, 16*(4), 17–26.

Marsella, A. J., & Christopher, M. A. (2004). Ethnocultural considerations in disasters: An overview of research, issues, and directions. *Psychiatric Clinics of North America, 27*(3), 521–539.

Masten, A. S., Hubbard, J. J., Gest, S. D., Tellegen, A., Garmezy, N., & Ramirez, M. (1999). Competence in the context of adversity: Pathways to resilience and maladaptation from childhood to late adolescence. *Development and Psychopathology, 11*, 143–169.

Ogbu, J. U. (1981). Origins of human competence: A cultural-ecological perspective. *Child Development, 52*(2), 413–429.

Sinha, J. B. P., & Kumar, R. (2004). Methodology for understanding Indian culture. *The Copenhagen Journal of Asian Studies, 19*, 89–104.

Suh, E. M., & Koo, J. (2008). Comparing subjective well-being across cultures and nations. In M. Eid & R. J. Larsen (Eds.), *The science of subjective well-being* (pp. 414–427). New York, London: The Guilford Press.

Tamis-LeMonda, C. S., Way, N., Hughes, D., Yoshikawa, H., Kalman, R. K., & Niwa, E. Y. (2008). Parents' goals for children: The dynamic coexistence of individualism and collectivism in cultures and individuals. *Social Development, 17*(1), 183–209.

Triandis, H. C. (1995). *Individualism & Collectivism*. Boulder, Oxford: Westview Press.

Triandis, H. C. (2004). The many dimensions of culture. *Academy of Management Executive, 18*(1), 88–93.

Triandis, H. C., & Suh, E. M. (2002). Cultural influences on personality. *Annual Review of Psychology, 53*, 133–160.

Uchida, Y., Norasakkunkit, V., & Kitayama, S. (2004). Cultural constructions of happiness: Theory and empirical evidence. *Journal of Happiness Studies, 5*, 223–239.

Van de Vliert, E., Schwartz, S. H., Huismans, S. E., Hofsteede, G., & Daan, S. (1999). Temperature, cultural masculinity, and domestic political violence. *Journal of Cross-Cultural Psychology, 30*(3), 291–314.

Chapter 3
Child Well-Being

Child Well-Being Indicator Movement

The research field of child well-being indicators originates from the so-called social indicators movement of the 1960s and 1970s following the long history of studying social trends (Ben-Arieh 2010; Fattore et al. 2007; Lippman 2007; Moore et al. 2008) as described above. The basic question of the social indicators research 'How are we doing?' is adapted to children—'How are our kids (including adolescents and youths) doing?' (Land et al. 2011).

> Indicators of child well-being are statistics that provide a sense of whether a group of children enjoy a good quality of life (O'Hare 2012, p. 79).

The use of child well-being indicators is manifold and they serve different purposes (Land et al. 2011; Moore 1999; Moore et al. 2003; O'Hare 2012): (1) *public attention*: a practical way to reach a broad audience, (2) *description*: to provide knowledge about society, (3) *setting goals*: to establish quantifiable thresholds to be met within a specific time period, (4) *outcomes-based accountability*: to measure and improve outcomes, (5) *monitoring*: to signal whether a group of children is moving in the right direction, and (6) *evaluation*: to determine whether programs are effective or not.

Recent Shifts in the Field of Child Well-Being Indicators

Research concerning the state of children has undergone several changes over time. Ben-Arieh (2010) identified nine major shifts from the focus of (1) child survival to child well-being, (2) negative to positive outcomes in life, (3) incorporating children's rights to looking beyond, (4) well-becoming to well-being, (5) indicators deriving from traditional domains to emerging indicators from new domains, (6) adults' to children's perspectives, (7) looking at national geographical units to measuring at a variety of geographical units, (8) a conceptual discussion of potential uses to policy orientation, and (9) increased supply of information to a composite index of child well-being.

Some of the shifts in the current child indicators movement met the requests of Orville Brim almost forty years ago. Brim (1975) demanded that new studies in this field have to address the questions on the child's subjective state, on the child's being and on the child's sense of self. Current indicators go beyond survival indicators, which measure mainly the fulfillment of basic needs; they measure the state and quality of life of children (e.g., their perceived notion of safety) (Ben-Arieh 2006; Ben-Arieh and Goerge 2001). Moreover, new indicators address child well-being from a child's perspective, rather than the well-becoming from an adult-centered perspective like the attainment of traditional age-based milestones (Lippman 2007). Also Brim's last request moving from traditional domains such as physical well-being and intellectual capacity to new domains including for example civic life skills is met (Ben-Arieh and Goerge 2001).

Out of these shifts in child well-being indicators identified by Ben-Arieh (2006, 2010), Fernandes et al. (2012) highlighted three trends in their review on child well-being measurements: (1) child-centered focus, (2) multi-dimensionality in child well-being, and (3) reliance on composite child well-being indices.

Child-Centered Focus

Within a child-centered approach, the child is the unit of analysis instead of the family or household where the child is integrated (Fernandes et al. 2012; Frones 2007).

Furthermore, there is a necessity of including children actively in the process of indicator development for measuring and monitoring their own well-being (Ben-Arieh 2005, 2006; Mason and Danby 2011). Taken into account the child's opinion in any matter affecting him or her is the fourth core principle of the UN Convention on the Rights of the Child (CRC) (Article 12: Respect for the views of the child). In general, numerous authors (Ben-Arieh 2005; Ben-Arieh 2010; Bradshaw et al. 2007) emphasize the importance of a child-rights-based approach in the development of child well-being indicators. Ben-Arieh (2005) argues that child well-being indicators, which are not—at least in part—gained from interactions with children, cannot claim to be based on the CRC.

Multi-Dimensionality in Child Well-Being

According to Bronfenbrenner's bioecological model of human development, children interact with their environment and play an active role in creating their well-being (Bronfenbrenner and Morris 2006). This ecological perspective emphasizes the multi-dimensionality of child well-being. Most scholars consider several indicators that reflect the different aspects of children's lives when analyzing how they are doing (e.g., Bradshaw et al. 2007; Land et al. 2007).

Composite Well-Being Child Indices

The growth on data on the construction of child well-being indicators is enormous (Ben-Arieh 2005; Frones 2007). Consequently, measures of overall child well-being have been developed using composite indices from a collection of indicators that cover a variety of domains, instead of measuring only one dimension of well-being (O'Hare and Gutierrez 2012; Lamb and Land 2013).

Well-Being Domains

Monitoring the situation of children is not new, and there are numerous reports on child well-being that have been published around the world since at least the 1960s (see Ben-Arieh and Goerge 2001 for a detailed literature review). An increase in the collection of social indicators related to children in order to capture the concept of well-being can be recorded over the past twenty years (Ben-Arieh and Frones 2007; O'Hare 2012).

> Child well-being encompasses quality of life in a broad sense. It refers to a child's economic conditions, peer relations, political rights, and opportunities for development. Most studies focus on certain aspects of children's well-being, often emphasizing social and cultural variations. Thus, any attempts to grasp well-being in its entirety must use indicators on a variety of aspects of well-being (Ben-Arieh and Frones 2007, p. 249).

According to the outcomes of an examination of 19 key studies, which combined domains into indices, there was little agreement on the number of domains that represented best a comprehensive composite child well-being index (O'Hare and Gutierrez 2012). However, the literature review indicated that nearly every study that involved a comprehensive composite child well-being index incorporated education, health, and material well-being domains into their index construction (ibid.). Ten years ago, in their literature review on child well-being—which did not focus on the use of domains within the context of comprehensive composite indices—Pollard and Lee (2003) identified five distinct well-being domains: physical, psychological, cognitive, social, and economical. Also Moore et al. (2011) state that common child well-being domains include physical, psychological, social, and educational/intellectual well-being. Those well-being domains directly assess how children are faring and are distinguished from contextual well-being, the characteristics of the child's environment that affect well-being (Moore et al. 2008, 2011).

In general, it is difficult to define what the key indicators of child well-being are, since personal values and definitions about children's well-being vary and underlie cultural forces (Fattore et al. 2009; Pollard and Lee 2003).

Composite Child Well-Being Indices

Table A.1 illustrates domains and indicators of composite child well-being indices, which incorporate the main trends in the field of child well-being indicators research identified by Fernandes et al. (2012) (see above). The choice of indices introduced in the table is based on what is considered in literature as some of the most relevant composite child well-being indices according to various scholars (e.g., Dex and Hollingworth 2012; Fernandes et al. 2012; Lamb and Land 2013; O'Hare and Gutierrez 2012). The first three indices are evidence-based national composite child well-being indices. The last three studies represent children's and young people's understanding of their own well-being and what accounts for a good life. The study of Gabhainn and Sixsmith (2005) was one (out of four) main component for the development of the national set of child well-being indicators in Ireland.

- Child and Youth Well-Being Index (CWI) (Land et al. 2001, 2007, 2011) for children and young people in the United states: 28 key indicators are compiled into seven domains.
- Index of Child Well-Being in Europe—EU 27 (Bradshaw and Richardson 2009), update of the EU 25 (Bradshaw et al. 2007): 43 indicators are combined into 19 components, which in turn are combined into 7 domains (components and domains are presented in Table A.1).
- National Survey of America's Families (NSAF)—Microdata Child Well-Being Index (Moore et al. 2007, 2008): Two composite indices—*child well-being index (individual)* with four domains, 16 subdomains, and 43 indicators; a *contextual well-being index* with three domains, 13 subdomains, and 26 indicators; parents are the respondents (domains and subdomains are presented in Table A.1).

The following indices involved children in defining their understanding of well-being:

- Children's Conceptualization of Their Well-Being in Australia (Fattore et al. 2007, 2009): 9 domains and 29 dimensions.
- Children's Understandings of Well-Being in Ireland (Gabhainn and Sixsmith 2005): 22 categories (the categories are presented in Table A.1, assignment to domains took place by the authors of the present book).

The goal of Andresen and Fegter (2011) study was to perform a systematic assessment of children's perspectives on a good life:

- Children's views on a good life—a childhood study in Germany (Andresen and Fegter 2011): six overall topics covering 'a good life' (overall topics are presented in Table A.1, assignment to domains took place by the authors of the present book).

Table A.1 (see Appendix) compiles indicators or components of well-being emerging from the studies listed above. A variety of ways to present the diverse sets of findings were considered. In the end, Dex and Hollingworth (2012) way of presenting was more or less followed. It was started with Land et al. (2011) work and successively the domains and indicators of the other authors were added. The list does not claim to be exhaustive or displayed in an accurate manner, but rather is intended to give a summary of child well-being indicators.

Purpose of the Present Study

The present study 'Development of child well-being indicators in South India (Tamil Nadu and UT Puducherry) after the 2004 Tsunami disaster' is part of the project 'Three years post-Tsunami: Long-term effects of trauma in children aged 7–15—A culture-sensitive approach,' which combined quantitative and qualitative methods to elicit trauma symptoms, behavior difficulties, and resources of children five years post-Tsunami.

A Culture-Sensitive Approach

Applying Western ways of categorizing psychiatric and or psychological states in different cultural contexts may have the effect that an assessment misses certain culture-specific ways of expressing and interpreting the world (De Silva 2006; Marsella and Christopher 2004; Summerfield 1999). Similarly, in order to obtain an understanding of the local factors, which constitute cultural valuable resources and well-being, it is necessary to step beyond Western notions of well-being by applying an approach that is sensitive toward contextual factors (Fattore et al. 2007, 2009). To meet the requirements of a culture-sensitive approach, the Inter-Agency Standing Committee (2007) requested in their guidelines on mental health and psychosocial support in emergency settings that the affected population should be actively involved in defining well-being and distress.

The purpose of the present study was to find out what makes up child well-being from a caregiver's and a child's perspective in the given subculture more than four years after the Tsunami disaster. Both, caregivers and children were given the opportunity to shape the well-being concept. McAuley and Rose (2010) argue that their (caregiver and children) involvement as key stakeholders guarantees that the discourse is grounded in reality.

Following an ecological perspective of human development (Bronfenbrenner and Morris 2006) as requested by various child well-being researchers (Bradshaw et al. 2007; Land et al. 2007; McAuley and Rose 2010), caregivers' and children's viewpoints—living in different social environments: fishing village versus SOS Children's Village—were contrasted. Moreover, the aim was not to produce an 'index of child well-being' for the Indian or even the Asian context. The idea was to document contextualized indicators of what it means for 'these' children in 'this' place to be doing well (or not) under the given circumstances (long-term effects in a post-disaster setting) (see also Crivello et al. 2009). The explicit aims were:

- to give children as well as their caregivers a voice in order to formulate in their own words what constitutes well-being for them
- to identify similarities and differences of mothers' concepts of well-being living in two different microsystems (fishing village vs. SOS Children's Village) as well as similarities and differences of children's concepts of well-being living in two different microsystems (fishing village vs. SOS Children's Village)
- to develop contextualized child well-being index—a culture-sensitive list for identifying children's well-being and ill-being from a child's perspective only.

References

Andresen, S., & Fegter, S. (2011). Children growing up in poverty and their ideas on what constitutes a good life: Childhood studies in Germany. *Child Indicators Research, 4*(1), 1–19.

Ben-Arieh, A. (2005). Where are the children? Children's role in measuring and monitoring their well-being. *Social Indicators Research, 74*, 573–596.

Ben-Arieh, A. (2006). *Measuring and monitoring the well-being of young children around the world*. Paper Commissioned for the EFA Global Monitoring Report 2007, Strong Foundations: Early Childhood Care and Education. http://unesdoc.unesco.org/images/0014/001474/147444e.pdf. Accessed June 9 2013.

Ben-Arieh, A. (2010). Developing indicators for child well-being in a changing context. In C. McAuley & W. Rose (Eds.), *Child well-being. Understanding children's lives* (pp. 129–142). London and Philadelphia: Jessica Kingsley Publishers.

Ben-Arieh, A., & Frones, I. (2007). Indicators of children's well-being: What should be measured and why? *Social Indicators Research, 84*, 249–250.

Ben-Arieh, A., & Goerge, R. (2001). Beyond the numbers: How do we monitor the state of our children? *Children and Youth Services Review, 23*(8), 603–631.

Bradshaw, J., & Richardson, D. (2009). An index of child well-being in Europe. *Child Indicators Research, 2*, 319–351.

Bradshaw, J., Hoelscher, P., & Richardson, D. (2007). An index of child well-being in the European Union. *Social Indicators Research, 80*, 133–177.

Brim, O. G. (1975). Childhood social indicators: Monitoring the ecology of development. *Proceedings of the American Philosophical Society, 19*(6), 413–418.

Bronfenbrenner, U., & Morris, P. A. (2006). The bioecological model of human development. In W. Damon & R. M. Lerner (Eds.), *Handbook of child psychology, theoretical models of human development* (6th ed., Vol. 1, pp. 793–828). New York: Wiley.

Crivello, G., Camfield, L., & Woodhead, M. (2009). How can children tell us about their well-being? Exploring the potential of participatory research approaches within young lives. *Social Indicators Research, 90*, 51–72.

De Silva, P. (2006). The Tsunami and its aftermath in Sri Lanka: Explorations of a Buddhist perspective. *International Review of Psychiatry, 18*(3), 281–287.

Dex, S., & Hollingworth, K. (2012). *Children's and young people's voices on their well-being.* Childhood Well-Being Research Centre, Working Paper 16. http://www.cwrc.ac.uk/documents/FINAL_Dex__September_2012__Report_on_childrens_voices_on_wellbeing_Working_Paper.pdf. Accessed June 9 2013.

Fattore, F., Mason, J., & Watson, E. (2007). Children's conceptualization(s) of their well-being. *Social Indicators Research, 80*, 5–29.

Fattore, F., Mason, J., & Watson, E. (2009). When children are asked about their well-being: Towards a framework for guiding policy. *Child Indicators Research, 2*, 57–77.

Fernandes, L., Mendes, A., & Teixeira, A. A. C. (2012). A review essay on the measurement of child well-being. *Social Indicators Research, 106*, 239–257.

Frones, I. (2007). Theorizing indicators. *Social Indicators Research, 83*, 5–23.

Gabhainn, S. N., & Sixsmith, J. (2005). *Children's understanding of well-being.* Centre for Health Promotion Studies, National University of Ireland. http://www.dcya.gov.ie/documents/research/childrenunderstandingofwellbeing.pdf. Accessed June 9 2013.

Inter-Agency Standing Committee (IASC). (2007). *IASC guidelines on mental health and psychosocial support in emergency settings.* Geneva: IASC.

Lamb, V.L., & Land, K.C., (2013). Methodologies used in the construction of composite child well-being indices. In A. Ben-Arieh (Ed.), *Handbook of child well-being.* New York: Springer. (http://www.soc.duke.edu/∼cwi/Section_I/I-17MethodologiesUsedinConstruction ofCompositeCWBIndices.pdf. Accessed June 9 2013).

Land, K. C., Lamb, V. L., & Mustillo, S. K. (2001). Child and youth well-being in the United States, 1975-1998: Some findings from a new index. *Social Indicators Research, 56*, 241–320.

Land, K. C., Lamb, V. L., Meadows, S. O., & Taylor, A. (2007). Measuring trends in child well-being: An evidence-based approach. *Social Indicators Research, 80*, 105–132.

Land, K. C., Lamb, V. L., & Zheng, H. (2011). How are the kids doing? How do we know? Recent trends in child and youth well-being in the United States and some international comparisons. *Social Indicators Research, 100*, 463–477.

Lippman, L. (2007). Indicators and indices of child well-being: A brief American history. *Social Indicators Research, 83*, 39–53.

Marsella, A. J., & Christopher, M. A. (2004). Ethnocultural considerations in disasters: An overview of research, issues, and directions. *Psychiatric Clinics of North America, 27*(3), 521–539.

Mason, J., & Danby, S. (2011). Children as experts in their lives: Child inclusive research. *Child Indicators Research, 4*, 185–189.

McAuley, C., & Rose, W. (2010). Child well-being: Current issues and future directions. In C. McAuley & W. Rose (Eds.), *Child well-being. Understanding children's lives* (pp. 207–218). London and Philadelphia: Jessica Kingsley Publishers.

Moore, K. A. (1999). Indicators of child and family well-being: The good, the bad and the ugly. *Child Trends*, Sept 13. http://www.childtrends.org/files/child_trends-1999_09_13_sp_indicatorscf.pdf. Accessed June 9 2013.

Moore, K. A., Brown, B. V., & Scarupa, H. J. (2003). The uses (and misuses) of social indicators: Implications for public policy. *Child Trends Research Brief*, 2003-1. http://www.childtrends.org/wp-content/uploads/2003/02/child_trends-2003_02_01_rb_useandmisuse.pdf. Accessed June 9 2013.

Moore, K. A., Vandivere, S., Lippman, L., McPhee, C., & Bloch, M. (2007). An index of the condition of children: The ideal and less-than-ideal U.S. example. *Social Indicators Research, 84*, 291–331.

Moore, K. A., Theokas, C., Lippman, L., Bloch, M., Vandivere, S., & O'Hare, W. (2008). A microdata child well-being index: Conceptualization, creation, and findings. *Child Indicators Research, 1,* 17–50.

Moore, K. A., Mbwana, K., Theokas, C., Lippman, L., Bloch, M., Vandivere, S., & O'Hare, W. (2011). Child well-being: An index based on data of individual children. *Child Trends Research Brief.* http://childtrends.org/wp-content/uploads/2013/03/ChildWellBeing.pdf. Accessed June 9 2013.

O'Hare, W. P. (2012). Development of the child indicator movement in the United States. *Child Development Perspectives, 6*(1), 79–84.

O'Hare, W. P., & Gutierrez, F. (2012). The use of domains in constructing a comprehensive composite index of well-being. *Child Indicators Research, 5,* 609–629.

Pollard, E. L., & Lee, P. D. (2003). Child well-being: A systematic review of the literature. *Social Indicators Research, 61,* 59–78.

Summerfield, D. (1999). A critique of seven assumptions behind psychological trauma programmes in war-affected areas. *Social Science and Medicine, 48,* 1449–1462.

Chapter 4
Development of Child Well-Being Indicators Four Years After the Tsunami Disaster

Method

The Tsunami Disaster

On December 26, 2004, a massive undersea earthquake off the west coast of northern Sumatra in Indonesia with a Richter-scale magnitude of 9.0 caused a giant Tsunami that devastated the shorelines of Indonesia, Sri Lanka, India, Thailand, and several other countries (International Centre for Migration and Health—ICMH 2005). No one knows exactly how many people lost their life in the Tsunami. The number of the dead and missing people varied depending upon the different sources. According to ICMH (2005), 180,000 people were estimated to have been killed. In India, the Union Territories of Andaman and Nicobar Islands and Puducherry (formerly known as Pondicherry) as well as the coastal areas of the states of Tamil Nadu, Kerala, and Andhra Pradesh were the most affected (United Nations, World Bank and Asian Development Bank 2006). But the worst damage was sustained in the state Tamil Nadu with a coastline of about 1,000 km and Andaman and Nicobar. In Tamil Nadu, 289 children were left as double orphans (Government of India and UNICEF 2005).

The whole study took place at Nagapattinam district, one of the most hit parts of Tamil Nadu and at the Union Territory Puducherry.

Participants and Setting

Participants were 112 Tsunami-affected children and their 56 caregivers. The children were either living with their biological parent(s) or in an alternative family-based out-of-home care. SOS Children's Village, which represents the alternative family-based out-of-home care in this study, is an independent non-governmental and social development organization. SOS Children's Villages operates worldwide in 133 countries and territories (SOS Children's Villages

S. Exenberger and B. Juen, *Well-Being, Resilience and Quality of Life from Children's Perspectives*, SpringerBriefs in Well-Being and Quality of Life Research, DOI: 10.1007/978-94-007-7519-0_4, © The Author(s) 2014

Table 4.1 Demographic characteristics of children participating in the focus groups according to age, sex, and location

Sex	Younger age group living in fishing village	Younger age group living in SOS CV	Older age group living in fishing village	Older age group living in SOS CV	Total
Female	14	12	23	13	62
Male	13	11	20	6	50
	27	23	43	19	**112**

International 2013) and focuses on children who lost parental care and/or children who are at risk to lose it (SOS Children's Villages International 2009). The organization pioneered a family approach to the long-term care of orphaned and abandoned children. Each child lives with a caring parent (SOS mother), with social and biological brothers and sisters in a house, within a SOS village (SOS Children's Villages International 2003). In India, there are 41 SOS Children's Villages across the country (SOS Children's Villages International 2013). Forty-two children of the present study lived either in SOS Puducherry or SOS Nagapattinam. Both villages came into existence a few years (2008 and 2007, respectively) after the Tsunami disaster (SOS Children's Village India 2013). Seventy children lived with their surviving parent(s) and came from two severely affected fishing villages of Nagapattinam district (Akkaraipettai and Keechankuppam) and two indirectly affected villages (Silladi of Nagapattinam district and Narambai in UT Puducherry). Fifty boys and 62 girls in the age range of 8 to 17 years took part in the study. The children were divided into two age groups: 'older girls/boys' (12 to 17 years) and 'younger girls/boys' (8 to 11 years). Table 4.1 gives an overview about the demographic characteristics of children. The group of caregivers was exclusively represented by mothers. Originally, some fathers could be recruited, but they stated that they were unable to give detailed information about their children and referred to their wives. However, fifteen SOS mothers and 41 mothers from the villages mentioned above represent the adult sample.

Procedure

Culture-Broker

From Pondicherry University, Department of Social Work, two students (male and female) for interpreting in same-sex groups were recruited for the entire research process. The students were selected according to the following criteria: *bi-lingual* (Tamil and English)—especially their spoken Tamil was of importance as in the Tamil language, there is a huge gap between spoken and written Tamil; *openness* to follow another approach in dealing with children without giving up their own cultural values; *consequence* and *perseverance* in the requested manner of interpreting. These two students acted as so-called culture-brokers—well-informed intermediaries whose inputs were brought to bear on the intervention process (Weidman 1975). A code of conduct was written concerning how to deal with the children (e.g., no punishment; self-determined working in small groups) and why the first author would like that they deal in that specific way with the children. The reasoning for this code was also interactively discussed with the interpreters. With regard to their specific task as interpreters, they were requested (1) to interpret in short units of meaning, (2) to avoid self-initiated interposed questions, (3) to avoid side-conversations with the children during the focus group sessions, (4) to participate in games and other relaxation exercises, and (5) to be confidential. In addition, they underwent a two-day training by the first author on the topics (1) family-based out-of-home care (SOS Children's Village), (2) different types of disasters and their impact, (3) trauma and well-being in children, (4) focus groups, and (5) transcription of audio material.

Focus Group Discussions

An applied qualitative methodology, that is focus group discussions as described by Lamnek (2005) for adults, and focus group discussions according to Vogl (2005) for children, was employed to gain understanding of well-being of directly and indirectly Tsunami-affected children. Before starting with the implementation of focus group discussions, informed consent was obtained of adults and children. The written informed consent was handed out approximately one week before the research started, and orally, confirmations about participation at the study were obtained. In addition, caregivers were asked for their agreement that their children take part in the research. A child-friendly version of an informed consent was repeated verbally at the beginning of focus group discussions. At any stage of the research process, each child as well as each caregiver was allowed to leave the group without giving any reason. Refusal of participation was rare.

To gain an understanding about what factors children identify as contributing to their well-being and ill-being, respectively, the *children* were asked the following main questions:

- What (in general) gives you happiness? What makes you happy?
- What makes you feel sad or unpleasant?
- If you feel sad or unpleasant, what helps you to feel good again?

The questions were chosen on the basis of Fattore et al.'s (2007) study findings, who asked children about their concept of well-being. 'Well-being is defined through feelings in particular happiness, but integrating sadness is also relevant' (Fattore et al. 2007, p. 18). Another reason to ask children about the causes for their happiness and sadness, respectively, was that they are supposed to understand these feelings easily, and in addition, it reflects the more operative construct of

SWB (Diener et al. 2003; Veenhoven 2008). The data of Harter's (1982) study demonstrated that already 3-year-olds clearly understood the feelings happy, sad, and mad and could consistently generate these three emotional labels.

The focus group discussions with children were initialized with an introduction game, followed by the orally obtained informed consent. The topic was introduced with a picture showing Indian children playing happily. Once the children had used the term 'happy' or 'happiness' in their description of the picture, the group discussion was opened with the first question. In a similar way the 'sad topic' was introduced. Both topics were discussed in small groups and afterward in the plenum. For the last question, the children were asked to use modeling clay or colors and paper to make a symbol of their coping strategy to come out of a sad or unhappy mood. Their symbols were discussed in the whole group. After each topic, a game was played. At the end of the focus group discussions drinks and snacks were provided to make sure that the children left the sessions in a happy mood. During snack time, the children had the possibility to ask questions or just to chat. In case a child got upset during the discussion process, he or she was supported to come out of his or her sad mood by the first author.

The focus group discussions with the caregivers were structured in a similar way, except there were no games during the course of group discussions and no prompting materials and mediums (picture, colors, modeling clay) were used. The caregivers were requested to answer the same questions as the children from their perspective. Just like the children, the caregivers answered the questions in small groups and discussed afterward their results with the whole group.

All focus groups were audio-taped. A focus group discussion with adults took about one hour. Two focus groups with SOS mothers (six and nine participants, respectively) and three focus group discussions per ten village mothers and one with twelve were implemented. The group discussions with children took up to two hours due to the involvement of play elements and working with different stimulating materials. Same-sex and same-age groups were formed. Each group consisted about a maximum of ten children. Five focus groups were implemented with SOS children in the facilities of SOS Children's Village where they lived. Additional eight groups with children from the fishing villages took place in community centers of the respective community where the children came from. All focus groups were conducted from February until April 2009. The cultural adequacy of the implementation process was guaranteed through the Indian supervisor of NIMHANS (see Chap. 1).

Data Preparation and Analysis

The Tamil answers of the recorded focus group discussions were translated into English. The transcribed interviews were analyzed on the basis of the qualitative research methodology 'grounded theory' (Glaser and Strauss 1967) which investigates the actualities in the real world and analyzes data with no preconceived hypothesis. In a first step, words and phrases of the interviewees that highlight an issue of importance or interest to the research are noted. Notes are generated and organized manually, for each descriptor phrase codes are assigned, and similarly, codes are grouped into so-called concepts (Corbin and Strauss 2008). In the present research, concepts are renamed into subcategories. These subcategories are then grouped and regrouped to find yet higher-order commonalities called categories. This is done by the constant comparative method (Glaser and Strauss 1967) that means each subcategory is compared to all other subcategories to form even broader categories. At a very high and abstract level of analysis, categories are bundled into core-categories, which are called 'domains' in this study. From a most abstract level of the analysis—the core-category—it is possible to go back (within the data pool) to the most basic group of data—the codes, which reflect the original phrases of the interviewees.

Results

The analysis of children's and mothers' transcribed focus group discussions resulted in the identification of five distinct domains, twelve categories, and fifty subcategories (Exenberger and Juen 2011). The data were quantified on a group level and not on the statements of an individual child or mother. That means, subcategories were only mentioned when one group of children or one group of mothers viewed them as important indicators for children's well-being. All domains consisted of positive and negative indicators referring to children's well-being and ill-being, respectively.

In the following, the data are presented in detail comparing the analysis of the two groups of mothers (mothers living in fishing villages versus SOS mothers) and the groups of children according to the context they live.

Domains, Categories, and Subcategories of Mothers Living in Fishing Villages Versus SOS Mothers

Table 4.2 shows domains, categories, and subcategories of mothers living in fishing villages (henceforward village mothers) compared to SOS mothers. The analysis of mothers' data living in fishing villages revealed five domains, eight categories, and fourteen subcategories. Out of the data of SOS mothers, three domains, five categories, and twelve subcategories were identified.

Table 4.2 Domains, categories, and subcategories of village mothers compared to SOS mothers

Mothers living in fishing villages			SOS mothers		
Domain	Category	Subcategory	Domain	Category	Subcategory
Cognitive	Academic	Future perspectives, school	Cognitive	Academic	School
Social	Appreciation	Appreciation of others	Social	Appreciation	Appreciation of self by others, of others
	Family	Parenting		Family-based out-of-home care	Attachment, parenting
	Peers	Play			
Psychological	Coping	Imagination, strategies of mothers to help children to cope with trauma	Psychological	Coping	Avoidance, distraction, support for emotional/instrumental reasons
	Tsunami-related symptoms	Triggers of feelings, impact of Tsunami, behavior of children/parents related to Tsunami, children's and adults' processing of Tsunami experience, memories		Tsunami-related symptoms	Triggers of feelings, impact of Tsunami, behavior of children/parents related to Tsunami, children's and adults' processing of Tsunami experience
Physical	Health	Health, accident, disaster-related needs/fears			
Economic	Materialism	Fulfillment of wishes			

Cognitive Domain

The cognitive domain consisted of one category, namely 'academic,' by both groups of mothers. Two subcategories were identified for the group of village mothers and one for SOS mothers. Village mothers mentioned as examples for children's ill-being, their low concentration in school, irregular attendance especially after Tsunami, and their little faith in future. SOS mothers emphasized as source of children's well-being that children were able to realize the importance of school and education for them.

> After Tsunami, nearly one year, the children did not go to school properly. Mostly due to fear they did not have proper attendance, and if they went, they also were full of fear when hearing small sounds (Village mothers).

Social Domain

For the group of village mothers, three categories with three corresponding subcategories could be identified. The categories comprised the topics 'appreciation,' 'family,' and 'peers.' The village mothers reflected the importance of appreciating other people, especially the mother. As their children did not appreciate their mothers since Tsunami, the mothers viewed this behavior as an indicator of their children's ill-being. Also the context in which mothers or widows had to raise their children was identified as a circumstance affecting their children's well-being negatively. Since their children's behavior toward peers has improved over the years after Tsunami, they clearly viewed this as a well-being indicator.

Two categories ('appreciation' and 'family-based out-of-home care') and four subcategories were found when analyzing the data of SOS mothers. The category 'appreciation' was broadened (when compared to the category 'appreciation' of village mothers) by the significance for the own person receiving appreciation of other people and consequently illustrated a source of children's happiness. The second category was a reflection of SOS mothers on their parenting style as it differed from the typical Tamil style of raising children. According to SOS mothers, this kind of parenting style contributed to children's ill-being on the long run.

> After Tsunami only, they are not listening our words. [...] Because they lost their father after Tsunami, my children do not respect me. They feel 'what can the mother do for me?' (Village mothers)

> If somebody said that sea water is coming, fear was there. But nowadays they are playing and they are good [with other children]. (Village mothers)

> ... one day, in a friendly manner, I [SOS mother] asked her [SOS child] 'why are you like this?' For that she [SOS child] replied 'I will do according to my wish only' ... So, we [SOS mothers] are not doing according to our wish, but to the wish of children only ... (SOS mothers)

Nowadays the girl is earning lot of fame from her class teachers and from other people who are there. (SOS mothers)

Psychological Domain

For the group of village mothers, the psychological domain comprised two categories, namely 'coping' and 'Tsunami,' with two and five subcategories, respectively. 'Coping' reflected mainly those strategies that demonstrated how mothers supported their children to overcome their trauma. According to the village mothers, their children's only coping strategy was 'imagination.' The village mothers clearly demonstrated that Tsunami-related issues like media rumors about another Tsunami or natural changes (e.g., high water level) triggered the fear of children—even at present. The negative impact of Tsunami (up to present) on the families' and consequently children's psychological, social, physical, and economical well-being was described extensively. The absence of trauma symptoms (e.g., clinging, sleep disturbances, triggers) was viewed as signs of children's well-being. Village mothers' and children's mutual processing of the traumatic experience was illustrated in a positive way of dealing with the trauma. The subcategory 'behavior of children/parents related to Tsunami' was partly viewed as a well-being and partly as an ill-being indicator. Children's (uncontrolled) memories of Tsunami were accompanied by feelings of loss and worries, and consequently named as a sign of ill-being.

The analysis of SOS mothers' data revealed the same two categories—'coping' and 'Tsunami'—as identified in the village mothers' data analysis. According to them, their children used three coping strategies to deal with their traumatic experiences. The subcategories 'avoidance' and 'distraction' are self-explanatory. All attempts of children to share their feelings and thoughts with others were summed up in the subcategory 'support for emotional reasons.' Seeking advice, assistance, or information was summarized in the subcategory 'support for instrumental reasons.' SOS mothers viewed all coping strategies of their children as signs of well-being. The same causes for children's ill-being (except 'memories') as mentioned by the village mothers were illustrated by SOS mothers.

We say, if Tsunami comes again, precautions will announce in time, so we can run away from this place, we will not die. A car will come and pick us up. So don't get afraid. (Village mothers)

[...] now they have changed. They are going to dance class, music class etc. [...] to get rid of their sorrows. (SOS mothers)

During the rainy season, sea tides will be more. By seeing that, children get afraid and force us to migrate from the place because they think that Tsunami occurs again. (Village mothers)

Some elders are doing their fishing business, and some children go and play there. (Village mothers)

For every Tsunami obituary day, all the people and children will gather together and go to the place with some candles and flowers, where memory hall was constructed for the people who lost their lives in Tsunami. (Village mothers)

Even now, children are troubled by dreams of Tsunami. (Village mothers)

Physical Domain

The physical domain was only mentioned by village mothers and consisted of one category—'health,' which in turn comprised one subcategory 'health/accident/disaster.' The subcategory was a source of children's ill-being and referred to physical impairments caused by the Tsunami from which the children still suffered up to the present moment.

From that shock the children have problem of bleeding through the nose; even now the problem continues. (Village mothers)

Economic Domain

Like the physical domain, the economic domain could only be identified in the group of village mothers. The category 'materialism' consisted of one subcategory labeled 'fulfillment of wishes.' The subcategory referred mainly to the disadvantaged circumstances mothers had to raise their children without a father.

[…] everyone of us lost the husband, no one has a father […] 'if my father was alive, he will buy and give a lot of things to me that I need, but my mother won't', they [the children] say […] (Village mothers)

Discussion of Mothers' Views on Their Children's Well-Being

The aim of the focus group discussions with mothers was to identify indicators of their children's well-being. But taking a close look at Table 4.2 and the subsequent result descriptions, it leaps to the eye that particularly village mothers revealed a lot about their own well-being or ill-being by identifying indicators of their children's well-being or ill-being (struggle with survival—see below). They mentioned only a few positive indicators, in contrast to the predominantly named negative indicators. The two mentioned positive well-being indicators of village mothers were their children's revival of play activities with other children and their coping strategy (imagination) to overcome their trauma. The remaining statements referred to their own (mothers') struggle with survival: economically, physically and as a single parent, which all together affected their children's well-being negatively and led to the listing of ill-being indicators. This fact is not surprizing taking into account that female widowhood puts Indian women at risk, particularly those from lower castes living in rural areas (Jensen 2005; Pincha 2008). Lower caste women in general and widows in particular get assigned with a lower status (Jensen 2005) and with a more limited access to resources (e.g., information, social networks, and influence) compared to men (Pincha 2008). Children, of course, were aware of their family status—living in a mother-headed household. Consequently, they did not pay the mothers the appropriate amount of respect, as it would be behooved in a collectivistic culture where respect and obedience toward elders is one of the highest values (Tamil-LeMonda et al. 2008). The missing appreciation of the mother was another named ill-being indicator. Moreover, the long-term consequences of trauma were described by measuring children's well-being through the absence of trauma symptoms (e.g., clinging, sleep disturbances). This fact suggested that recovery from trauma was decelerated due to persistent chronic problems of living. That recovery processes are slowed down through lack of resources in developing countries is a well-known finding of trauma research (Neuner et al. 2006; Norris et al. 2002b; Pynoos et al. 1993). One group of village mothers expressed their misery with the following words:

> If Tsunami comes again, it should not leave one person and take another person of a family, it should take everyone from a family.

A hierarchial multiple regression analysis computed with data of the post-Tsunami project strongly substantiated the qualitative data suggesting mothers' ill-being strongly affects children's well-being in a negative way. The final model of the hierarchial multiple regression analysis showed that general health of the mothers estimated through the General Health Questionnaire (GHQ-28, Goldberg et al. 1997) ($\beta = 0.46$, $p < 0.001$) significantly predicted the amount of post-traumatic stress symptoms in children as did the context (fishing village versus SOS Children's Village) in which the children lived ($\beta = -0.18, p < 0.05$); living in a fishing village was a significant predictor for PTSD symptomatology.

Turning to the identified child well-being indicators of SOS mothers, it emerged that the statements of SOS mothers also referred to negative indicators, but their remarks were compensated with positive ones. Just as village mothers, SOS mothers measured their children's well-being in the absence of trauma symptoms. But they considered a child was doing well, when he or she realized the importance of education, got praised by others, could build up an attachment, and used a variety of coping strategies in order to come out of an unhappy mood. Extremely interesting was the fact that they did not mention any physical or economic well-being indicators. As these two well-being domains are used in the vast majority of child well-being indices according to O'Hare and Gutierrez (2012). One reason could be, that SOS mothers, even though some of them were widows or divorced—actually marginalized persons that would put them and their children in care at risk (Jensen 2005)—they felt 'on the safe side' as the organization is taking care of them and their children. But from the viewpoint of village mothers, it became very clear that well-being strongly depends on material well-being and health. They show a constant concern for survival as poverty can have a damaging effect on families through child labor and lack of children's social participation (Camfield 2012). According to Camfield (2012), access to material and social resources are necessary pathways to well-being. In terms of Cummins (2000), whenever the threshold for adaptation to negative life circumstances is exceeded, these difficult objective circumstances of living begin to drive SWB down.

Domains, Categories, and Subcategories of Children Living in Fishing Villages Versus SOS Children

Table 4.3 shows domains, categories, and subcategories of children living in fishing villages (henceforward: village children) compared to SOS children. The analysis of all children's data resulted in five domains and eleven categories. The two groups of children differed from each other in the amount of subcategories. For the group of village children 43 and for the group of SOS children 33, subcategories could be identified.

Cognitive Domain

The cognitive domain comprised one category 'academic' and three subcategories—'arts,' 'future perspectives,' 'school'—by both groups of children. The category 'academic' is mainly intellectual or school-related in nature. Expressing themselves artistically in the form of dance, drawing, singing, etc., scoring good marks in school, and consequently getting a positive outlook were sources of all children's happiness.

> Here [at SOS Children's Village] there are more activities which develop our skills. Also I like dance very much here. I get an opportunity to learn dance. (SOS children)

> If I don't go to school, I will be sad. (Village children)

> Going to computer class makes us happy. That will be very useful for us while doing our higher education. (Village children)

> Studying well is good for us and also for my mom [SOS mother]. If I study well, I will buy saree for my mom. (SOS children)

Table 4.3 Domains, categories, and subcategories of village children compared to SOS children

Children living in fishing villages			SOS children		
Domain	Category	Subcategory	Domain	Category	Subcategory
Cognitive	Academic	Arts, future perspectives, school	Cognitive	Academic	Arts, future perspectives, school
Social	Appreciation	Appreciation of self by others, appreciation of others, (in)justice, punishment	Social	Appreciation	Appreciation of self by others, (in)justice, punishment, reputation
	Civic life	Celebrating festivals, community life, cultural norms, political interest/interest in world affairs, religious life		Civic life	Celebrating festivals, political interest/interest in world affairs
	Family	Joint family, nuclear family, obedience, parenting		Family-based out-of-home care	Attachment, biological family, nuclear family, obedience
	Peers	Friends, competition, play		Peers	Friends, competition, play
	Social skills	Empathy, openness, pro-social behavior		Social skills	Empathy, openness, pro-social behavior
Psychological	Coping	Avoidance, belief, distraction, imagination, nature, pos. reinterpretation and growth, seeking support for emotional/instrumental reasons, support by others, self-blame, ventilation	Psychological	Coping	Belief, distraction, nature, pos. reinterpretation and growth, seeking support for emotional/instrumental reasons, support by others, ventilation
	Nature	Appreciation of environment, of nature		Nature	Appreciation of environment, of nature
	Tsunami-related symptoms	Behavior of children/parents related to Tsunami, children's and adults' processing of Tsunami experience, impact of Tsunami, memories, triggers of feelings		Tsunami-related symptoms	Impact of Tsunami, memories
Physical	Health	Health, accident, disaster-related needs and fears physical activities	Physical	Health	Health, accident, disaster-related needs and fears physical activities
Economic	Materialism	Fulfillment of wishes	Economic	Materialism	Fulfillment of wishes

Social Domain

Within the social domain, the categories 'appreciation,' 'civic life,' 'family' and 'family-based out-of-home care' (SOS children), respectively, and 'social skills' could be identified for both groups of children. All children mentioned the sub-categories 'appreciation of self by others' as source of happiness, and 'injustice' as well as 'punishment' (scolding and beating) as ill-being indicators. The subcategory 'appreciation of others' as a sign of one's own well-being was only mentioned by village children, and having a good reputation ('reputation') as source of happiness was solely named by SOS children. The subcategories 'friends,' taking part in competitions, e.g., singing competition, and 'play' were part of the category 'peers' and contributed to all children's well-being. As another source of happiness, all children named the category 'social skills' consisting of the subcategories 'empathy' (e.g., to be delighted in somebody else's happiness), 'openness' (e.g., to be interested in new people), and 'pro-social behavior.' All children stated that 'celebrating festivals' (diwali, birthday, etc.) make them feel happy, whereas national and international news, for example, the atrocities of the civil war in Sri Lanka, makes them feel sad ('political interest/interest in world affairs'). The subcategories 'community life,' 'religious life,' and 'cultural norms' concerned 'civic life' and were mentioned by the village children. 'Cultural norms' were considered as a source of unhappiness as often they had a restricting effect on the children. Being with the 'joint or nuclear family' and being 'obedient' in the sense of receiving good advice were contributing to village children's well-being. 'Parenting' was viewed negatively (by village children) when their parents or mothers demanded to do hard work in order to help them. All those subcategories counted among the category 'family.' The SOS children's subcategories slightly differed. For them, building an 'attachment' with the SOS mother was an indicator of well-being, and once this attachment was established, they enjoyed to be with their 'nuclear (SOS) family.' Meeting their 'biological family' was a source of happiness as well as receiving advice (subcategory 'obedience').

> Beating the children makes us feel unhappy. Parents are beating us. It is not good. (Village children)

> Some programs organized in our street we like very much. Panchayat [local government—wise and respected elders] organize programs like singing competition, dancing competition etc. We participate in that and have fun. (Village children)

> Here some people are staying in our village for laying roads. If we speak with them, all of our village mates scold us. (Village children)

> If we were been given hard work like carrying heavy weights, we feel sad. We cannot carry, but we have to carry for parents. (Village children)

> Going to functions like earring ceremony, marriage functions etc. gives us happiness. At such functions only we would be able to meet all our relatives (Village children)

When somebody calls us 'orphan', we turn around and say 'we are not orphan, we have mother, brother and sister'. (SOS children)

If they [friends] smile and feel happy, and me, I also feel happy then. (SOS children)

Psychological Domain

The categories 'coping,' 'nature,' and 'Tsunami-related symptoms' are summarized in the psychological domain. The first two categories contributed to all children's happiness, whereas the last category was a source of children's unhappiness. The coping strategies 'imagination' (only village children), 'seeking support for emotional/instrumental reasons,' and 'support by others' were already described above (result description of mothers). All children used the coping strategies 'belief' (e.g., praying), 'distraction,' 'nature' (e.g., looking at something beautiful in nature), 'positive reinterpretation and growth' (e.g., reflecting on own mistakes) and 'ventilation' (e.g., crying and feeling better afterward) to come out of their sorrows. In addition, village children coped with unpleasant situations by 'avoiding' them or 'self-blame.' The importance of 'nature' for all children emerged out of the data so that a separate category was formed. Both groups of children highly appreciated the beauty of nature ('appreciation of nature') in general and viewed the preservation of nature, taking care of the environment in particular as source of their well-being. Whereas Tsunami-related issues like 'memories' of Tsunami and the 'impact of Tsunami' in a psychological, social, physical, and economic point of view were (still—four years post-Tsunami) strong sources of all children's ill-being. Village children mentioned as an additional indicator of their ill-being that rumors about another Tsunami or high water levels triggered bad feelings ('triggers of feelings'). The two subcategories 'behavior of children/parents related to Tsunami' and 'children's and adults' processing of Tsunami experience' were both named as well-being as well as ill-being indicators solely by village children (see result description of mothers).

> When I feel sad, I look at flowers. In those flowers, I am able to see my father's face. He loved flowers. Also I am able to see my relatives' face, so I like flowers. And clouds. After the funeral of my father, they made many flowers in that place [...] (SOS children)
> When I am sad, I will think about the sun, because the sun is giving light to all, why can't I be like that. (SOS children)
> Rain. I like rain very much. Whenever it rains, I take a bath in the rain. (Village children)
> If plants or leaves become dry then I feel sad. Because trees help us in many ways, they give medicine, fruit etc. (SOS children)
> When the wastes are not disposed properly, it spreads many diseases to all the people. (Village children)

Physical Domain

The physical domain, which was mentioned by both groups of children, comprised one category with two corresponding subcategories: 'health/accident/disaster' (see result description of mothers) and 'physical activities.' While the first subcategory was a sure indicator for children's ill-being, the second was indicating children's well-being.

> Because of Tsunami all my family members died such as our dad, mom, siblings. That makes us sad. (SOS children)
>   In school we feel happy during physical education period. [...] They will provide volley ball (Village children).

Economic Domain

The fifth and last domain is the economic one. Village children as well as SOS children viewed the presence or absence of materialistic resources either con-tributing to their well-being or to their ill-being. The corresponding subcategory was labeled 'fulfillment of wishes.'

> We didn't get food. After we came here [SOS Children's Village] we are fine. Whatever we want, our mom [SOS mother] will get for us. Our mom is treating us well. (SOS children)
>   After school we are working. We must help our parents to repay their loans. (Village children).

Discussion of Children's Views on their Own Well-Being

The focus group discussions with children were attempted to uncover children's understanding of their well-being within their social contexts and in the given subculture. Some categories with their corresponding subcategories contributing to children's well-being were identical in both groups of children, some similar and some differed from each other showing the strong influence of ecology on a micro-level according to Bronfenbrenner's bioecological model of child development (Bronfenbrenner and Morris 2006). Identical subcategories or indicators were found in the following domains and categories: (1) 'cognitive/academic,' (2) 'social/peers,' (3) 'social/social skills,' (4) 'psychological/nature,' (5) 'physical/ health,' and (6) 'economic/materialism.' Similar subcategories or indicators could be identified in the domains and corresponding categories 'social/family' and 'psychological/coping.' The viewpoints of the two groups of children differed in the domains and corresponding categories 'social/civic life' and 'psychological/ Tsunami-related symptoms' (see also Exenberger and Juen 2010).

Both groups of children wanted to succeed when they are grown-up. They knew that they need good education for career advancement, which in turn they need to look after their own (future) family in a proper way as well as to support their family of origin. These high ambitions were clear indicators for child well-being as a 'foreshortened future' is quite common among traumatized children (Fletcher 2007).

In various studies, children highlighted the significance of family and peer relationships as well-being indicators (e.g., Andresen and Fegter 2011; Dex and Hollingworth 2012 for a review, Gabhainn and Sixsmith 2005). Also in the present investigation, positive relationships with their nuclear family (that is the biological family of village children and the SOS family of SOS children) and joint family as well as with peers accompanied by good experiences with them in competitions and play were mentioned by both groups of children as sources of happiness. SOS children experienced the SOS family especially positively, when they were able to establish an attachment with their SOS mother. The quality of parent–child relationship has far reaching consequences for a child's development. It predicts later social competence that in turn sets the course for positive (adjustment) or negative (maladjustment) developmental pathways (Werner 1993).

Even though the children of the present study listed a variety of coping strategies contributing to their well-being, different kinds of social support were emphasized. In general, social support has been identified as one of the most important resources for children in dealing with life stressors (Bolton et al. 2004). It appears that different people in children's lives offer different types of social support, and these various types of support may fulfill specific needs following disasters (Juen et al. 2004). For example, caregivers support children in the form of reinstituting familial roles and routines in the aftermath of disaster (Dyregrov 2008; Prinstein et al. 1996). Non-kin support such as friends have mediated the impact of disaster stress on depressive symptomatology in post-flood victims (Kaniasty and Norris 1993). In the long-term study of Bolton et al. (2004), the importance of friendship was highlighted even five to eight years post-event. Recovered survivors had higher functioning in the domain of friendship when compared with the control group. In general, mutual friendship and peer rejection are of great significance for later positive adult adjustment in different life domains (Bagwell et al. 1998). Not only receiving support mitigated children's sorrows but also the child's active approach to others, which also demonstrated the findings of Bolton et al.'s (2004) study. With regard to coping strategies, village children mentioned two additional strategies, namely 'avoidance' (e.g., avoiding places that trigger sad feelings) and 'self-blame' ('Even though Tsunami hit me, I should have saved my mom and sister. My sister is small, at least she might live good after that'—village children). It is not surprising that only village children named these rather negative coping strategies as they needed to recover from trauma in their destroyed villages of origin. The ongoing exposure to a number of traumatic reminders in the aftermath of disaster slowed down the recovery process (Pynoos et al. 1993), a fact that also has been noticed by village mothers. This could be an explanation that children draw on these less effective coping strategies. While avoidance strategies might provide temporary relief, in the long term, it worsens the problem because it prevents the memory from being fully processed (Smith et al. 2002). That the experience of Tsunami was not forgotten or fully worked through at least by village children illustrates Table 4.3. In contrast to SOS children, who relived their trauma in the past, the village children relived their trauma in the present. Even though village children related much more ill-being indicators to the incident, they also mentioned some well-being indicators in this regard. Due to the limited opportunities to avoid the stimuli associated with the trauma, village children counted triggers among their ill-being indicators, on the one hand. On the other hand, they also could recognize their own and parents' behavioral changes back to normality. For example, they dared to play alone next to the sea and their parents allowed them to do so. They also viewed positively their inclusion in activities and rituals related to the death of loved ones. Taking part in rituals and prayers can help children to find expression in feelings and to find closure for important events and troublesome thoughts (Dyregrov 2008). Rituals were of special importance in various Tamil communities after Tsunami as survivors had a tendency to collectivize their personal sorrows and consequently used collectively rituals as spiritual coping strategies (Rajkumar et al. 2008). Just as village children, SOS children were troubled by Tsunami-related memories, in particular, that due to Tsunami, they lost their family and had to remain in out-of-home care. Even though many SOS children valued their life at SOS Children's Village for the experiences and opportunities offered to them (e.g., proper food and education), yet they wished for their life with their own parents or at least for a life in their community. The category 'civic life' was the second category in which divergent results concerning the two groups of children were found. Village children reported about active participation in community and religious life that strongly contributed to their well-being. Even though, SOS children celebrated festivals just as village children and viewed this as source of happiness, they did not mention being part of community life. According to Morgan (2009), children in care stated that the longer they spend in care, the higher the risk of losing contact with birth family and friends, which can lead to feelings of unhappiness.

Both groups of children also mentioned social skills like 'empathy,' 'openness,' and 'pro-social behavior' contributing to their well-being. Especially after a disaster, these skills are clear indicators of increasing well-being as trauma disrupts the development of empathy and pro-social behavior (Osofsky 1995 in Lubit et al. 2003). 'Openness' in the sense of being happy to be confronted with new people, places, and situations signifies a child's interest to explore, which in turn shows that a child feels safe and has overcome trauma as clinging behavior often is a result of trauma (Lubit et al. 2003; Math et al. 2006).

Social relationships do not only increase children's sense of well-being, but also can significantly contribute to their ill-being (Dex and Hollingworth 2012; Thoilliez 2011). In the present study, both groups of children expressed that punishment, in form of beating and scolding by parents, teachers, and other significant adults, clearly contributed to their ill-being. Even though in the Tamil culture, physical affection for children is expressed more often than not by slaps, pinches, and tweaks (Trawick 1990) and children tried to reinterpret it positively, they unmistakably perceived punishment as source of unhappiness. One village girl stated: 'And I feel sad when my mother scolds me, but I don't take that as much serious as it is a quite normal thing that our mothers will scold. Our mothers will scold only for good sake.'

Although children listed numerous coping strategies to overcome their sorrows, one coping strategy 'nature' so strongly emerged in both groups of children that a separate same-named category within the psychological domain was formed. Nature was highly valued by the children, on the one hand as source for relaxation, on the other hand for clearing the mind. This finding is actually not surprising taking into account that meditation, yoga, and tantric healing practices are indigenous traditional psychological therapies in India (Bhatia 2006). In addition, children demonstrated remarkable environmental moral values and knowledge. They believed that, for example, trees were important for their lives and viewed pollution as source of ill-being. They were aware that for their future life, they would need a healthy environment, which again showed that those children's concept of their well-being was characterized by great diversity. These children— regardless of their personal faith—had a drive to succeed and to beat the odds.

References

Andresen, S., & Fegter, S. (2011). Children growing up in poverty and their ideas on what constitutes a good life: Childhood studies in Germany. *Child Indicators Research, 4*(1), 1–19.

Bagwell, C. L., Newcomb, A. F., & Bukowski, W. M. (1998). Preadolescent friendship and peer rejection as predictors of adult adjustment. *Child Development, 69*(1), 140–153.

Bhatia, S. (2006). Reinterpreting the inner self in global India: "Malevolent mothers", "distant fathers" and the development of children's identity—Review essay. *Culture and Psychology, 12*(3), 378–392.

Bolton, D., O'Ryan, D., Udwin, O., Boyle, S., & Yule, W. (2004). The long-term psychological effects of a disaster experienced in adolescence II: General psychopathology. *Journal of Child Psychology and Psychiatry, 45*(5), 1007–1014.

Bronfenbrenner, U., & Morris, P. A. (2006). The bioecological model of human development. In W. Damon & R. M. Lerner (Eds.), *Handbook of child psychology, theoretical models of human development* (6th ed., Vol. 1, pp. 793–828). New York: Wiley.

Camfield, L. (2012). Resilience and well-being among urban Ethiopian children: What role do social resources and competencies play? *Social Indicators Research, 107*, 393–410.

Corbin, J., & Strauss, A. (2008). *Basics of qualitative research* (3rd ed.). London: Sage Publications.

Cummins, R. A. (2000). Objective and Subjective quality of life: An interactive model. *Social Indicators Research, 52*, 55–72.

Dex, S., & Hollingworth, K. (2012). *Children's and young people's voices on their well-being.* Childhood Well-Being Research Centre, Working Paper 16. http://www.cwrc.ac.uk/documents/FINAL_Dex__September_2012__Report_on_childrens_voices_on_wellbeing_Working_Paper.pdf. Accessed 9 June 2013.

Diener, E., Oishi, S., & Lucas, R. E. (2003). Personality, culture, and subjective well-being: Emotional and cognitive evaluations of life. *Annual Review of Psychology, 54*, 403–425.

Dyregrov, A. (2008). *Grief in young children. A handbook for adults.* London: Jessica Kingsley Publishers.

Exenberger, S., & Juen, B. (2010). Post-Tsunami: The influence of context on children's subjective well-being. *Journal of the Indian Academy of Applied Psychology, 36*(2), 207–213.

Exenberger, S., & Juen, B. (2011). Four years post-Tsunami: Children's well-being. *Psychology Research, 1*(3), 193–202.

Fattore, F., Mason, J., & Watson, E. (2007). Children's conceptualization(s) of their well-being. *Social Indicators Research, 80*, 5–29.

Fletcher, (2007). Posttraumatic stress disorder. In E. J. Mash & R. A. Barekley (Eds.), *Assessment of childhood disorders* (pp. 398–483). New York: Guilford Press.

Gabhainn, S. N., & Sixsmith, J. (2005). *Children's understanding of well-being.* Centre for Health Promotion Studies, National University of Ireland. http://www.dcya.gov.ie/documents/research/childrenunderstandingofwellbeing.pdf. Accessed 9 June 2013.

Glaser, B., & Strauss, A. (1967). *The discovery of grounded theory.* Chicago: Aldine.

Goldberg, D. P., Gater, R., Sartorius, N., Ustun, T. B., Piccinelli, M., Gureje, O., et al. (1997). The validity of two versions of the GHQ in the WHO study of mental illness in general health care. *Psychological Medicine, 27*, 191–197.

Government of India and UNICEF's Tsunami Recovery Programme. (2005). Building back better for children. http://www.unicef.org/india/Tsunami_Book_Final.pdf. Accessed 9 June 2013.

Harter, S. (1982). A cognitive-developmental approach to children's understanding of affect and trait labels. In F. C. Serafica (Ed.), *Social-cognitive development in context* (pp. 27–61). New York: The Guilford Press.

International Centre for Migration and Health (ICMH). (2005). The public health consequences of the Tsunami: Impact on displaced people. http://www.icmhd.ch/publications_2005.htm. Accessed 9 June 2013.

Jensen, R.T. (2005). Caste, culture, and the status and well-being of widows in India. In D.A. Wise (Ed.), *Analyses in the economics of aging* (pp. 357-375). University of Chicago Press. http://www.nber.org/chapters/c10366. Accessed 9 June 2013.

Juen, B., Werth, M., Roner, A., Schönherr, C., & Brauchle, G. (2004). *Krisenintervention bei Kindern und Jugendlichen* (2nd ed.). Innsbruck: STUDIA Universitätsverlag.

Kaniasty, K., & Norris, F. H. (1993). A test of the social support deterioration model in the context of natural disaster. *Journal of Personality and Social Psychology, 64*(3), 395–408.

Lamnek, S. (2005). *Gruppendiskussion. Theorie und Praxis* (2nd ed.). Weinheim: Beltz Verlag.

Lubit, R., Rovine, D., Defrancisci, L., & Eth, S. (2003). Impact of trauma on children. *Journal of Psychiatric Practice, 9*(2), 128–138.

Math, S. B., Girimaji, S. C., Benegal, V., Kumar, G. S. U., Hamza, A., & Nagaraja, D. (2006). Tsunami: Psychosocial aspects of Andaman and Nicobar Islands. Assessments and intervention in the early phase. *International Review of Psychiatry, 18*(3), 233–239.

Morgan, R. (2009). *Keeping in touch.* London: Children's Rights Director, Ofsted. http://www.ofsted.gov.uk/resources/keeping-touch. Accessed 9 June 2013.

Neuner, F., Schauer, E., Catani, C., Ruf, M., & Elbert, T. (2006). Post-Tsunami stress: A study of posttraumatic stress disorder in children living in three severely affected regions in Sri Lanka. *Journal of Traumatic Stress, 19*(3), 339–347.

Norris, F. H., Friedman, M. J., & Watson, P. J. (2002b). 60000 disaster victims speak: Part II. Summary and implications of the disaster mental health research. *Psychiatry: Interpersonal and Biological Processes*, 65(3), 240–260.

O'Hare, W. P., & Gutierrez, F. (2012). The use of domains in constructing a comprehensive composite index of well-being. *Child Indicators Research, 5*, 609–629.

Pincha, C. (2008). *Indian Ocean Tsunami through the gender lens—Insights from Tamil Nadu, India.* Mumbai: Earthworm Books published for Oxfam America & NANBAN Trust.

Prinstein, M. J., La Greca, A. M., Vernberg, E. M., & Silverman, W. K. (1996). Children's coping assistance: How parents, teachers and friends help children cope after a natural disaster. *Journal of Clinical Child Psychology, 25*(4), 463–475.

Pynoos, R. S., Goenjian, A., Tashjian, M., Karakahian, M., Manjikian, R., Manoukian, G., et al. (1993). Post-traumatic stress reactions in children after the 1988 Armenian earthquake. *British Journal of Psychiatry, 163*, 239–247.

Rajkumar, A. P., Premkumar, T. S., & Tharyan, P. (2008). Coping with the Asian Tsunami: Perspectives from Tamil Nadu, India on the determinants of resilience in the face of adversity. *Social Schience and Medicine, 67*, 844–853.

Smith, P., Dyregrov, A., & Yule, W. (2002). *Children and disaster—Teaching recovery techniques*. Bergen: Children and War Foundation.

SOS Children's Village India. http://www.soschildrensvillages.in/where-we-work/Pages/default.aspx. Accessed 9 June 2013.

SOS Children's Villages International. http://www.sos-childrensvillages.org/Where-we-help/Asia/India/Pages/default.aspx. Accessed 9 June 2013.

SOS Children's Villages International (2003). *Who we are*. http://www.sos-childrensvillages.org/About-us/Publications/SOSwork/Documents/101206-WhoWeAre-en-WEB.pdf. Accessed 9 June 2013.

SOS Children's Villages International (2009). *SOS Children's Village Programme Policy*. http://www.sos-childrensvillages.org/About-us/Our-Approach/Documents/Programme-Policy-en-small.pdf. Accessed 9 June 2013.

SOS Children's Villages International (2011). *Facts and figures 2011*. http://www.sos-childrensvillages.org/About-us/Publications/Reports-studies/Documents/SOS-Facts-and-Figures-2011-EN-WEB.pdf. Accessed 9 June 2013.

Tamis-LeMonda, C. S., Way, N., Hughes, D., Yoshikawa, H., Kalman, R. K., & Niwa, E. Y. (2008). Parents' goals for children: The dynamic coexistence of individualism and collectivism in cultures and individuals. *Social Development, 17*(1), 183–209.

Thoilliez, B. (2011). How to grow up happy: An exploratory study on the meaning of happiness from children's voices. *Child Indicators Research, 4*(2), 323–351.

Trawick, M. (1990). *Notes on love in a Tamil family*. Berkeley: University of California Press.

United Nations, World Bank, and Asian Development Bank (2006). *Tsunami. India—Two years after*. Chennai, New Delhi: Author.

Veenhoven, R. (2008). Sociological theories of subjective well-being. In M. Eid & R. J. Larsen (Eds.), *The science of subjective well-being* (pp. 44–61). New York: The Guilford Press.

Vogl, S. (2005). Gruppendiskussion mit Kindern: Methodische und methodologische Besonderheiten. In Zentralarchiv für Empirische Sozialforschung (Ed.), *ZA-Information 57* (pp. 28–60). Köln: Universität zu Köln.

Weidman, H. (1975). Concepts as strategies for change. *Psychiatric Annals, 5*, 312–314.

Werner, E. E. (1993). Risk, resilience, and recovery: Perspectives from the Kauai longitudinal study. *Development and Psychopathology, 5*, 503–515.

Chapter 5
Children's Voices on Their Well-Being: A Child Well-Being Index

Method

Out of the concepts of mothers' and children's own views on child well-being, a list of child well-being indicators with 72 items was derived. With this index, the well-being of the children in the given subculture was measured.

Participants

Co-workers of the SOS Children's Village Nagapattinam recruited additional families (in addition to the focus group participants) that were affected by Tsunami and lived in the Nagapattinam district. Consequently, participants were 167 mothers who gave answers for their 344 children. Ninety-one mothers who lived with their Tsunami-affected children in fishing villages of Nagapattinam district (Akkaraipettai and Keechankuppam) gave answers for 179 children. Fifteen SOS mothers from the SOS Children's Villages Nagapattinam and Puducherry answered for 42 Tsunami-affected children in their care. All SOS mothers as well as 19 mothers of the fishing villages already took part in the focus groups discussions described above. The two students who already were interpreting during these discussions identified a local NGO, which operated in Periyapet, Puducherry district for recruiting non-Tsunami-affected families. With their help, 61 mothers could be engaged in order to complete the questionnaire for their 123 children. They were chosen according to the following criteria: similar living standard compared to the living standard of the fishing families, living away from sea, non-Tsunami-affected and living with at least two children aged 7–17 years in one household. Their children faced various adverse situations like the loss of a caregiver due to an accident, domestic violence, injuries, and different other accidents (e.g., fire). Mothers of Tsunami-affected children and mothers of non-Tsunami-affected children estimated the well-being with the developed child well-being index of approximately two of their children. SOS mothers answered questions about more children, depending on how many Tsunami-affected children lived in their SOS family. The mean age of children at the time of data collection was 11.7 years (SD 2.87, range 7–17 years). Information was available for 182 girls (mean age 11.6, SD 2.79, range 7–17 years) and 162 boys (mean age 11.8, SD 2.96, range 7–17 years).

Measure

Child well-being index. The original list of child well-being indicators (Exenberger and Juen 2011) comprised 72 statements concerning the well-being of children who have faced an adverse situation. The list of indicators is a culture-sensitive approach for the indication of child well-being in the given subculture. Mothers' as well as children's concepts of child well-being were reflected in this list. Children's well-being was assessed by caregiver reports on a 4-point response format (not true, little true, somewhat true, and true). The list is available in English and Tamil.

Procedure

Data were collected during May and October 2009. The developed list of child well-being indicators was part of a questionnaire battery concerning mothers' own (mental) health status and resources as well as their children's resources and mental health status. One session took up to two hours. The questionnaires were administered orally on an individual basis by four students. In addition to the two students (male and female student) who already were engaged as interpreters during the focus group discussions, two other female students from the same department were recruited. All four students got background information on all measures used. They also received training by the first author on (a) the understanding of the content of each questionnaire, (b) how to implement a questionnaire, (c) code of conduct that gave an explanation about how to deal with the participants during a session, and (d) the obtaining of the informed consent in an oral form. With role-play, the students practiced the procedure. During the recruitment process of mothers, oral informed consent was obtained. The study participants were not requested to sign as they felt uncomfortably giving their signature. However, a written version of the informed consent was distributed. Once date and time, place and transport were arranged, always two sessions were held parallel. All mothers of Tsunami-affected children (including SOS mothers) were questioned at the SOS Children's Village Nagapattinam. Mothers of the non-Tsunami-affected children were met at a center of the cooperating local NGO in Periyapet, Puducherry district. The first author was on site for opening the session and psychologically support if needed during or after a given session. At the beginning of each session, informed consent was repeated for the purpose of making rapport. Once the participant felt comfortably, each question was read aloud and an adjuvant answering sheet was applied. The questions were conducted in Tamil. All mothers received lunch during their session and had the possibility to rest. At the end, they received school material for their children as remuneration worth 100 rupees (equal to 1.50 Euro). The necessity for school material was identified by a co-worker from SOS Children's Village Nagapattinam.

Data Preparation and Analysis

All data were analyzed by using SPSS 16.0 software. The original list of 72 items was reduced to 64 statements as mothers' concepts of well-being were completely reflected in children's concepts. Consequently, the 64 statements display exclusively children's own concepts of their well-being and were derived from children affected by the Tsunami disaster (see description above).

A principal component analysis (PCA) was conducted on 64 items (children's concepts of well-being) with orthogonal rotation (varimax). The Kaiser–Meyer–Olkin (KMO) measure was used to assess sampling adequacy. With Bartlett's test of sphericity, it was calculated whether the correlation matrix was significantly different from an identity matrix. An initial analysis was run to obtain eigenvalues for each component in the data. Cronbach's alpha (α) was used to measure scale reliability.

Results

Factor Structure

To identify the factor structure of the children's concept of well-being, a PCA was conducted on 64 items with orthogonal rotation (varimax). The values of 0.71 for the KMO measure of sampling adequacy for the analysis indicated that the proportion of variance in the variables was caused by underlying factors. According to Kaiser (1974, cited in Field 2009, p. 647), this value was above the acceptable limit of 0.5. Furthermore, Hutcheson and Sofroniou (1999) considered values between 0.7 and 0.8 as good. Thus, it allowed for the application of factor analysis. This was supported by the Bartlett's test of sphericity $\chi2$ (2016) = 6580,584, $p < 0.001$, indicating that correlations between items were sufficiently large for PCA. An initial analysis was run to obtain eigenvalues for each component in the data. As twenty components had eigenvalues over Kaiser's criterion of 1, the analysis was rerun. Seven factors were specified to be extracted, and in combination they explained 38.3 % of the variance. The items that clustered on the same components suggested that *component* 1 represents (absence of) other trauma-related symptoms, *component* 2 academic achievement, *component* 3 (absence of) trauma-related fears and intrusions, *component* 4 coping, *component* 5 community orientation, *component* 6 (absence of) fear of punishment, and *component* 7 family compliance.

Reliability

For all 64 items, Cronbach's alpha was 0.78. Regarding the seven subscales, Cronbach's alpha for the '(absence of) other trauma-related symptoms' items was 0.72, for the 'academic achievement' items was 0.82, for the '(absence of) trauma-related fears and intrusions' items was 0.80, for the 'coping' items was 0.62, for the 'community orientation' items was 0.73, for the '(absence of) fear of punishment' items was 0.57, and for the 'family compliance' items was 0.39. According to Kline (1999), values for Cronbach's alpha of 0.7–0.8 are acceptable values, and even values below even 0.7 can realistically be expected when dealing with psychological constructs. While the components 1, 2, 3, and 5 had high reliabilities, the components 4 and 6 had relatively low and the component 7 extremely low reliability.

Table 5.1 shows the factor loadings after rotation, eigenvalues, percentage of variance that each factor explains and the reliability analysis.

Description of Components

After conducting factor analysis, the complete list of child well-being indicators consisted of forty items. Items that clustered on the same components suggested that *component* 1 consisted of seven items, which represented (absence of) other

Table 5.1 Summary of exploratory factor analysis results for the list of child well-being indicators according to children's concepts (N = 290)

	Rotated factor loadings						
	(Absence of) other trauma-related symptoms	Academic achievement	(Absence of) trauma-related fears and intrusions	Coping strategies	Community orientation	(Absence of) fear of punishment	Family compliance
Eigenvalues	6.22	4.48	4.25	3.26	2.39	2.04	1.86
% of variance	6.40	6.22	6.00	5.93	5.41	4.23	4.07
α	0.72	0.82	0.80	0.62	0.73	0.57	0.39

trauma-related symptoms. That means the child maintains positive relations with siblings as well as peers and feels comfortable at home. The child himself or herself is no bullying victim. The *second component* was academic achievement with five items: the child is aware of the importance of studies for his or her future, shows good results in academics, and has concrete future plans. *Component* 3 concerned (absence of) trauma-related fears and intrusions and consisted of seven items. The child does not suffer from intrusive memories and avoidance symptoms. Fear or negative feelings are not triggered when the child is confronted with various reminders of Tsunami. The child has taken up activities that he or she enjoyed already before Tsunami (e.g., taking a bath in sea). Coping strategies was the leading topic of *component* 4 comprising seven items. Nature, support by friends, and distraction are the prominent coping strategies. *Component* 5, community orientation, was made up of seven items. In general, this component combines activities, which include mainly non-family members just as friends or peers. Examples are taking part in programs organized in the streets, showing the own talents in competitions, going on tour. The (absence of) fear of punishment was represented in *component* 6 with four items. Sources of fear of punishment are beating, scolding, and bad news on an international and national level. Family compliance consisting of three items constituted the last component. Following advices of parents, going to the temple, and concerns about the environment are the topics of this component.

Discussion

A PCA was conducted with 64 statements which were derived exclusively from children's concepts of their well-being. Seven factors could be identified (see Table 5.1), where of four factors concerned children's well-being and three factors children's ill-being. All factors more or less reflected the domains and categories of children's views on their well-being and ill-being, respectively, derived from the qualitative data (see Table 4.3). The ill-being factors were reformulated in a positive way.

The first domain 'absence of trauma-related symptoms' mainly summarized the maintenance of and the integration into peer relationships as well as positive relationships within the nuclear family. The occurrence of these trauma-related symptoms indicated that the child has not overcome his or her trauma yet. In general, social withdrawal, problematic social relationships, and increased aggressiveness are clear symptoms of trauma in school-age children and adolescents (Lubit et al. 2003; Williams 2006). The domain 'absence of trauma-related fears and intrusions' contained primarily characteristics of a posttraumatic stress disorder (PTSD) symptomatology according to DSM-IV (American Psychiatric Association 1994). Items concerning avoidance of places, intrusive distressing recollections of the event, etc., were included in this domain. The third ill-being domain 'absence of fear of punishment' comprised on the one hand parenting techniques like beating and scolding, on the other hand bad national and international news which triggered generalized anxiety.

The four well-being domains were characterized consistently by a strong social component. In collectivism, the self is not viewed as separated from the social context, but as very much connected. It implies that group membership is central to identity and well-being derives from successfully carrying out social roles and obligations (Markus and Kitayama 1991). For example, academic achievement did not only comprise academic success like scoring good marks, but also a good relationship with the teacher. Apart from the importance of nature as a preferred coping strategy, emphasis was put on social relationships in the domain 'coping.' Interaction with others either on an individual or on group basis was summarized in the domain 'community orientation.' The factor 'family compliance' mainly reflected obedience, for example, whether the child followed advices or not.

The physical as well as the economic domain did not cluster on a separate component. Both domains were implicitly reflected in other domains. For example, the wish to succeed in academics and future perspectives were not meant for individual career development, but in order to take care for caregivers later on. The health domain was strongly related to healthy caregivers who could provide adequate care for the children. Consequently, when the basic needs more or less are fulfilled children do not mention explicitly the need for material and health security. The same was true for SOS mothers (see Table 4.2) who did not indicate health and economic indicators as they and their children received a high level of care.

Table 5.2 shows the summary of contextualized well-being indicators from the viewpoint of children. In this table, the subcategories are divided into objective and subjective indicators. Objective indicators reflect an external measurable perspective, and subjective indicators mirror an internal one that only can be experienced by the individual himself or herself. The number of domains was reduced to the essential: social, psychological, and cultural domain. The cognitive, economic, and health domains, which originally were identified by children and village mothers in the qualitative data (but not in the quantitative, at least economic and health did not cluster on separate components), were assigned to the social domain. This strongly reflects a child perspective on well-being as not the own health but the health of others is emphasized as well as the material well-being was mentioned mainly in connection with the whole family. The cultural indicators strongly reflect the context the children live in and place special emphasis on collectivist values.

Wellness is an ecological concept; a child's well-being is determined by the level of parental, familial, communal, and social wellness (Prilleltensky and Nelson 2000, p. 87).

As we mentioned before, child well-being can only be fully understood when integrating the three concepts of well-being, quality of life, and resilience. Furthermore, our study showed the multidimensional characteristics of all three concepts. Figure 5.1 depicts our theoretical model toward a full understanding of child well-being highlighting the three identified dimensions in each concept.

Table 5.2 Summary of results

Domain	Category	Subcategory—objective indicators	Subcategory—subjective indicators
Social	Academic achievement	Academic achievement: school attendance, school achievement	Subjective meaning of academic achievement: being able to take care of family, future perspective, appreciation of self by praise of teachers, relationship with teachers
	Quality of family/ parenting	Nuclear family, contact to biological family, availability of caregivers, supportive behavior of caregivers, social network, lack of domestic violence	Perception of parenting styles: obedience, feeling of safety against domestic violence, attachment to caregivers
	Peer relationships	Peer relationships: having friends, playing with other children	Perception of peer relationships, open for play and joyful playing
	Health of others	Physical health: objective health of child and caregiver	Physical health: feeling healthy, caregiver's health
	Material well-being for family	Economic resources, standard of living (housing)	Feeling of safety, future orientation—caring for family
Psychological	Appreciation	Appreciation of self: reputation and status	Feeling accepted by others
	Social skills	Openness, pro-social	Empathy, openness
	Coping skills and trauma coping	Coping skills: not too much avoidance behavior, distraction behavior, going out to nature, talking to others about negative experiences, seeking support for emotional and instrumental reasons	Coping skills: imagination of positive outcome, positive reinterpretation of negative experiences, posttraumatic growth, lack of self-blame, reintegrating memories, affective regulation of negative feelings
Cultural	Appreciation of nature	Taking care of nature and environment, going into nature	Love for nature, feeling/ enjoying the calming effect of nature
	Community orientation	Competitive games, taking part in community activities	Loving community activities
	Arts activities	Taking part in arts activities	Loving arts activities
	Joint family	Having a joint family and being part of it, having a community and being part of it	Feeling of embeddedness in joint family, feeling of embeddedness in community
	Obedience	Lack of punishment, respect for elders (gender issues: respect for mother even though no father)	Respect for elders (gender issues: respect for mother even though no father)

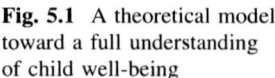

Fig. 5.1 A theoretical model toward a full understanding of child well-being

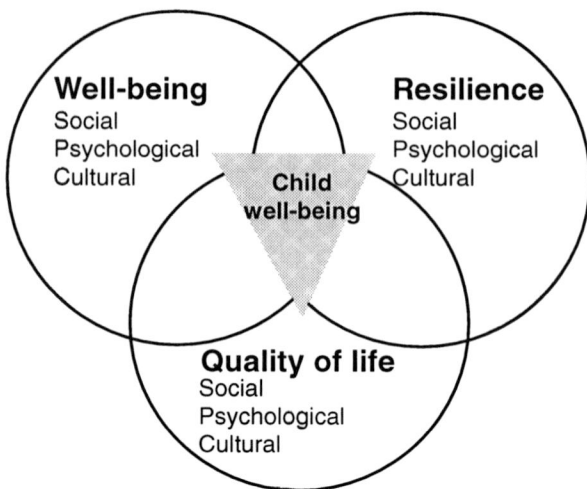

Dimension 1 is the social domain (e.g., objective—school achievement, and subjective—being able to take care of the family in future), *dimension* 2 the psychological domain (e.g., objective—reputation, and subjective—feeling accepted by others), and *dimension* 3 the cultural domain (objective—going into nature, and subjective—feeling/enjoying the calming effect of nature).

References

American Psychiatric Association. (1994). *Diagnostic and statistical manual of mental disorders* (4th ed.). Washington, DC: Author.

Exenberger, S., & Juen, B. (2011). Four years post-Tsunami: Children's well-being. *Psychology Research, 1*(3), 193–202.

Field, A. (2009). *Discovering statistics using SPSS* (3rd ed.). London: SAGE Publications.

Hutcheson, G., & Sofroniou, N. (1999). *The multivariate social scientist*. London: SAGE Publications.

Kline, P. (1999). *The handbook of psychological testing* (2nd ed.). London: Routledge.

Lubit, R., Rovine, D., Defrancisci, L., & Eth, S. (2003). Impact of trauma on children. *Journal of Psychiatric Practice, 9*(2), 128–138.

Markus, H. R., & Kitayama, S. (1991). Culture and the self: Implications for cognition, emotion and motivation. *Psychological Review, 98*(2), 224–253.

Prilleltensky, I., & Nelson, G. (2000). Promoting child and family wellness: Priorities for psychological and social interventions. *Journal of Community and Applied Social Psychology, 10*, 85–105.

Williams, R. (2006). The psychosocial consequences for children and young people who are exposed to terrorism, war, conflict and natural disasters. *Current Opinion in Psychiatry, 19*, 337–349.

Chapter 6
Conclusions

This research was one work-package of a larger project and provided an account of children's as well as their mothers' understanding of what constitutes child well-being in the long-term aftermath of the Indian Ocean Tsunami in Tamil Nadu and UT Puducherry, India. The study participants were Tsunami-affected mothers who lived with their children in fishing villages, non-Tsunami-affected SOS mothers and their Tsunami-affected children in care. This specific work-package aimed to meet the general request of various scholars (IASC 2007) to actively involve the affected population in defining their well-being and distress. Four important conclusions referring to the composition of children's well-being have emerged from the present research and are presented in the subsequent sections:

1. *Mothers' well-being needs to be secured in order to enable children's well-being.*

The impact of Tsunami became very clear through the village mothers' estimation about how they viewed that their children were doing well. During the focus group discussions, village mothers mainly referred to their own ill-being due to their widowhood and their economic struggle with survival as a consequence thereof. It is a well-known fact in trauma research that children's well-being and recovery from trauma strongly depend on their caregiver's well-being and their dealing with the trauma (Dyregrov 2006; Lustig et al. 2004). Material security is one indispensable pathway to well-being [see Camfield (2012)] as once the threshold for adjustment to negative life circumstances is exceeded, well-being is negatively affected (Cummins 2000). The findings of the present study revealed that lack of economic resources had far-reaching consequences by also affecting children's social well-being. For example, village children reported that due to their bad economic circumstances, they were partly socially excluded (e.g., they could not join small trips organized by school) and temporarily could not attend school because of workloads at home. Another consequence of mothers' ill-being was their reduced resources to spend time with their children. When they described how they could see that their children were doing well, they mainly noticed the decrease in trauma symptoms as children's posttraumatic stress symptoms were a

big burden in their survival struggle: 'For us, we get food only when we work. We
go to business at 2 a.m. and children get afraid to be alone. They won't allow us to
go to work' (village mothers). They did not recognize the variety of children's
manifold resources and coping skills that constitutes child well-being. That
became very clear when contrasting mothers' child well-being concepts with that
of children's; no additional well-being indicator was listed which has not already
been covered by the children themselves.

2. *Disasters enable and promote social change.*

Sekar et al. (2005) distinguished different natures of impact due to a disaster:
physical, economic, emotional, and social. Within the social domain, basic
structures such as family, living, and community structures get affected. For
children, especially the changes in family structure due to the loss of family
members are crucial. In the present study, they revealed how hard they tried to
pave the way for a better future life for themselves and their family. But their
efforts more or less remained unnoticed. They hardly could bear the injustice of
punishment (beating and scolding) anymore. They 'requested'—to express it in a
provocative way—for new strategies of teaching and parenting. This request
confronted a guiding child-rearing principle in Tamil Nadu: Downgrading the
loved one, and the containment of love (or anpu—how it is called in Tamil),
especially the love of the mother, which is the most crucial one (Trawick 1990).
To come back to the overstress of village mothers and the resulting lack of time
recognizing their children's resources (as outlined above), it becomes an imperative to sensitize caregivers for recognizing their children's resources. When
considering the Whitings hypothesis that changes in parenting are brought about
more by socioeconomic and population changes than the introduction of new
ideologies (Edwards and Bloch 2010), a chance for change could become reality.
The resilience building program of Exenberger et al. (2010) was on the one hand
aimed to sensitize caregivers for children's resilience, on the other hand to build
resilience in children.

3. *Importance of social relationships and enabling of new relationships and
   networks after disaster.*

The findings of various studies on child well-being indicated that social relations to family and friends are exceptionally important to most children (e.g.,
Andresen and Fegter 2011; Fattore et al. 2009; Gabhainn and Sixsmiths 2005).
Also in the present study, this result was strongly confirmed and even extended to
the larger context, namely the community the children belong to. Not only in the
immediate but also in the long-term aftermath of disasters social resources appear
to be extremely vulnerable as disasters remove significant supporters from survivors' networks through death (Norris et al. 2002a). In addition, temporary or
permanent relocation challenges the survivors' social abilities to build up new
social networks. The successful establishment of attachment to a new caregiver

contributed significantly to SOS children's well-being. They fended potential bullies off (getting bullied for being an orphan) by telling them that they live in a family. The interpersonal relationships of children participating in the present study were of great importance for their well-being as how well they were doing depended to a large extent on the quality and strength of their social network [see also Crivello et al. (2009)]. This already implies not only the family contributed to children's happiness, but also the larger social context like their community. In estimating their happiness, collectivists do not refer to their own mental state, but to their social network (Triandis 1999). At this point, the impact of collectivist values on the meaning of well-being emerges. In the present study, it was of immense importance for the children being an active part of their community and being part of community rituals to overcome the long-term effects of Tsunami. In the aftermath of disaster, the community plays a crucial role in preventing a possible social collapse. The response is often that a collective is coming together to rebuild and reaffirm the collective identity (Marsella and Christopher 2004). A collective identity (the feeling of belonging on a micro- as well as macro-level) contributes crucially to children's happiness. Evans (2005) labeled a socially and materially rich environment as 'social resilience.' Children cannot be resilient by only relying on their individual strengths they also need access to (material and social) resources (Ungar 2005, 2008), especially in a collectivistic culture, in which individualistic values like self-esteem are not very helpful. According to Camfield (2012), the strengths of people children relate to may be as important in their resilience as their own characteristics. This implies that not only the children need to be strengthened in post-disaster settings, but also their close and wider social context in order to promote their resilience which in turn enables them to positive well-being outcomes.

4. *The imperative of defining cultural child well-being indicators.*

As already outlined above, well-being is being used widely and in very different ways. According to Ereaut and Whiting (2008), well-being is a cultural construct and subject to shifting meanings. It depends on what groups of people collectively agree makes 'a good life.' Well-being is subject to culture. Joshanloo (2013) criticizes the current literature on happiness and well-being as it either takes a culture-free stance or is rooted in Western streams of thought. The present study clearly pointed out the importance of and need for contextualized indicators, which reflect the given subculture. On the one hand, already well-known well-being indicators implicated a different cultural meaning, and on the other hand completely new indicators were named by the children. For example, children's academic achievement was driven by their wish to succeed in order to support their family of origin. Children somehow agreed to the claim of their caregivers to grant old-age security [see also Aycicegi-Dinn and Kagitcibasi (2010)], but they also wanted to show their gratitude and make them happy. Their wish to attend activities organized by the community—for example competitions where children had the chance to show their talents—illustrated their need for a strong, healthy, and active community, which gives them the possibility to participate. Contrariwise, the community needs strong, healthy, and active children because they are vital to the social and economic recovery for a community and on a large scale for a country after a disaster (Goenjian et al. 2001). In terms of Prilleltensky and Nelson (2000), it can be said that mainly collectivist values in this study characterized the identified well-being indicators of children. Collectivist values are those that strive to enhance the well-being of the community at large (ibid.).

One of the most striking findings of the present study was that the sight of beauty—mainly something in nature such as a flower, the shape of clouds—helped the children to gain inner peace and helped them to overcome sorrows. Among hectic and crowd, children were able to create their own inner private psychological space where they could back down for a few moments to reload their strengths and overcome sorrows. This inner self is a highly protected reservoir for their inner needs and ambitions and enables them to become individuated (Sinha et al. 2001) in a collectivist surrounding. The individual benefit of this secret space is well known by the children as source of happiness. The high value of this inner space expressed their wish for nature preservation and the children also wished to share their good spirit (which reminds to the eudaimonic approach of happiness) with others by making flower presents. According to Prilleltensky and Nelson (2000), the most interventions serve individual goals in order gain well-being, and rather neglect collectivist goals, but the promotion of collectivist values is crucial as a strong community is vital in supporting individuals to achieve their goals. 'Nature' contributing to children's happiness was a cultural and very new indicator—when compared to other study results, which aimed to identify well-being indicators (see Table A.1). Against the background of a Hindu doctrine, the indicator 'nature' is not surprising, but a highly valuable indication toward calming and cure in the aftermath of disaster. '[…] true joy comes from contentment and peace of mind brought about by constantly acknowledging that in everything dwells the Supreme Being (Brahman)' (Joshanloo 2013). In Hinduism, the key ingredients of a good life are the practice of virtues and a contended state of mind (Joshanloo 2013).

The book is closing with placing a special emphasis on the indispensable value on children's perspectives on their well-being. It follows the trends on child well-being measurements identified by Fernandes et al. (2012): (1) child-centered focus, (2) multidimensionality, and (3) composite child well-being indices. The documentation of contextualized indicators, of what it means for these children in this place at this point of time—in the long-term aftermath of the Tsunami disaster—reflects children's views on what constitutes a 'good life' in its sovereignty.

Acknowledgments The research leading to these results has received funding from the European Community's Seventh Framework Programme FP7-PEOPLE-2007-4-1-IOF, Marie Curie Actions—International Outgoing Fellowships (IOF) under grant agreement no. 220535.

We would like to thank all children and mothers for their enthusiastic and valuable contributions during the focus group discussions. We also would like to acknowledge the invaluable support of SOS Children's Villages India, particularly Mr. Siddharta Kaul—current President of SOS Children's Villages International. We are grateful to the research team in India who contributed in very significant ways to the study described here: R. Kumuthavalli and G. Vijai Amirtharaj.

References

Andresen, S., & Fegter, S. (2011). Children growing up in poverty and their ideas on what constitutes a good life: Childhood studies in Germany. *Child Indicators Research, 4*(1), 1–19.

Aycicegi-Dinn, A., & Kagitcibasi, C. (2010). The value of children for parents in the minds of emerging adults. *Cross-Cultural Research, 44*(2), 174–205.

Camfield, L. (2012). Resilience and well-being among urban Ethiopian children: What role do social resources and competencies play? *Social Indicators Research, 107*, 393–410.

Crivello, G., Camfield, L., & Woodhead, M. (2009). How can children tell us about their wellbeing? Exploring the potential of participatory research approaches within Young Lives. *Social Indicators Research, 90*, 51–72.

Cummins, R. A. (2000). Objective and subjective quality of life: An interactive model. *Social Indicators Research, 52*, 55–72.

Dyregrov, A. (2006). A review of PTSD in children. *Child and Adolescent Mental Health, 11*(4), 176–184.

Edwards, C. P., & Bloch, M. (2010). The Whitings' concepts of culture and how they have fared in contemporary psychology and anthropology. *Journal of Cross-Cultural Psychology, 41*(4), 485-498.

Ereaut, G., & Whiting, R. (2008). *What do we mean by 'wellbeing'? And why might it matter?* Research Report DCSF-RW073. London: Department for Children, Schools and Families.

Evans, R. (2005). Tanzania. Social networks, migration, and care in Tanzania. Caregivers' and children's resilience to coping with HIV/AIDS. *Journal of Children and Poverty, 112*, 111–129.

Exenberger, S., Juen, B., & Sekar, K. (2010). *Resilience building among children in adverse situations.* Innsbruck: University of Innsbruck, Department of Psychology (internal publication).

Fattore, F., Mason, J., & Watson, E. (2009). When children are asked about their well-being: Towards a framework for guiding policy. *Child Indicators Research, 2*, 57–77.

Fernandes, L., Mendes, A., & Teixeira, A. A. C. (2012). A review essay on the measurement of child well-being. *Social Indicators Research, 106*, 239–257.

Gabhainn, S. N., & Sixsmith, J. (2005). *Children's understanding of well-being.* Centre for Health Promotion Studies, National University of Ireland. http://www.dcya.gov.ie/documents/research/childrenunderstandingofwellbeing.pdf. Accessed 9 June 2013.

Goenjian, A. K., Molina, L., Steinberg, A. M., Fairbanks, L. A., Alvarez, M. L., Goenjian, H. A., Pynoos, R. S. (2001). Posttraumatic stress and depressive reactions among Nicaraguan adolescents after Hurricane Mitch. *American Journal of Psychiatry, 158*, 788–794.

Inter-Agency Standing Committee (IASC). (2007). *IASC guidelines on mental health and psychosocial support in emergency settings.* Geneva: IASC.

Joshanloo, M. (2013). Eastern conceptualizations of happiness: Fundamental differences with Western views. *Journal of Happiness Studies.* doi:10.1007/s10902-013-9431-1.

Lustig, S., Kia-Keating, M., Grant-Knight, W., Geltman, P., Ellis, H., Birman, D., Kinzie, D., Keane, T., and Saxe, G. (2004). Review of Child and Adolescent Refugee Mental Health. *Journal of the American Academy of Child and Adolescent Psychiatry, 43*(1), 24–36.

Marsella, A. J., & Christopher, M. A. (2004). Ethnocultural considerations in disasters: An overview of research, issues, and directions. *Psychiatric Clinics of North America, 27*(3), 521–539.

Norris, F. H., Friedman, M. J., & Watson, P. J. (2002a). 60000 disaster victims speak: Part I. An empirical review of the empirical literature, 1989–2001. *Psychiatry: Interpersonal and Biological Processes, 65*(3), 207–239.

Prilleltensky, I., & Nelson, G. (2000). Promoting child and family wellness: Priorities for psychological and social interventions. *Journal of Community and Applied Social Psychology, 10*, 85–105.

Sekar, K., Bhadra, S., Jayakumar, C., Aravindraj, E., Henry, G., & Kishorekumar, K. V. (2005). *Psychosocial care in disaster management.* Bangalore: NIMHANS.

Sinha, J. B. P., Sinha, T. N., Verma, J., & Sinha, R. B. N. (2001). Collectivism coexisting with individualism: an Indian scenario. *Asian Journal of Social Psychology, 4*, 133–145.

Trawick, M. (1990). *Notes on love in a Tamil family.* Berkeley: University of California Press.

Triandis, H. C. (1999). Cross-cultural psychology. *Asian Journal of Social Psychology, 2*, 127–143.

Ungar, M. (2005). Pathways to resilience among children in child welfare, corrections, mental health and educational settings: Navigation and Negotiation. *Child and Youth Care Forum, 34*(6), 423–444.

Ungar, M. (2008). Resilience across cultures. *British Journal of Social Work, 38*, 218–235.

Appendix

S. Exenberger and B. Juen, *Well-Being, Resilience and Quality of Life*
from Children's Perspectives, SpringerBriefs in Well-Being and Quality of Life Research,
DOI: 10.1007/978-94-007-7519-0, © The Author(s) 2014

Table A.1 Domains and indicators of evidence-based national composite well-being indices and child well-being indices from children's points of view (a selection)

	CWI (Land et al. 2001, 2007, 2011)	EU27 (Bradshaw and Richardson 2009)	NSAF – Microdata (Moore et al. 2008)	Fattore et al. (2009)	Gabhainn and Sixsmith (2005)	Andresen and Fegter (2011)
Material well-being	X	X	X (sociodemographic context)	X		
Poverty rate/enough material resources	x	x	x	x	x	
Secure parental employment rate	x	x				
Median annual income	x		x			
Health insurance coverage	x		x (family context)			
Deprivation		x				
Human capital			x		x	
Family size			x		x	
Money					x	
Technology					x	
Food					x	x
Social relationships (social health—Moore et al. 2008)	X	X	X (individual)	X (Dealing with adversity)	X	
Single-parents headed families	x		x (family structure—sociodemogr.)			
Moved within the last year	x					
Quality of family relationships	x	x	x	x	x	x
Peer relationships	x	x	x	x	x	x

(continued)

Table A.1 (continued)

	CWI (Land et al. 2001, 2007, 2011)	EU27 (Bradshaw and Richardson 2009)	NSAF – Microdata (Moore et al. 2008)	Fattore et al. (2009)	Gabhainn and Sixsmith (2005)	Andresen and Fegter (2011)
Adults outside family				x		x
Solve problems				x		
Strategies to relieve from stress				x		
Positive social behaviors		x				
Negative social behaviors		x				
Pets					x	x
Opposite sex					x	
To be loved and cared						x
Somebody to love						x
Physical closeness						x
(Physical) health	**X**	**X**	**X (individual)**	**X**		
Infant mortality rate	x	x				
(Low birth) weight rate	x	x	x			
Mortality rate	x	x (risk and safety)				
Overweight children and adolescents	x					
Overall health status	x		x	x		
Activity limitation	x					
Immunization		x				
Health behavior/healthy lifestyle		x	x	x	x	
Access to health services				x		x
Chronic health condition			x			

(continued)

Table A.1 (continued)

	CWI (Land et al. 2001, 2007, 2011)	EU27 (Bradshaw and Richardson 2009)	NSAF – Microdata (Moore et al. 2008)	Fattore et al. (2009)	Gabhainn and Sixsmith (2005)	Andresen and Fegter (2011)
(Psychological) health			**X (individual)**			
Internalizing problems			x			
Externalizing problems			x			
Coping skills			x			
Safety/risk/behavioral concerns	**X**	**X**		**X**		
Teenage birth rate	x	x				
(absence) of violence	x	x		x		x
Violence crime offenders	x	x				
Health risk behavior	x	x	x (health)			
Feeling safe at home				x		
Child friendly communities				x		
Productivity (educational attainment)	**X**	**X**	**X (individual)**			
Reading test scores	x	x				
Mathematics test scores	x	x				
Outcomes		x				
Learning difficulties			x			
Cognitive development			x			
Achievement			x			
School					x	x
School pressure						x
Activities, freedom, competence, fun				**X**		
Enjoy experience of learning				x	x	x

(continued)

Table A.1 (continued)

	CWI (Land et al. 2001, 2007, 2011)	EU27 (Bradshaw and Richardson 2009)	NSAF – Microdata (Moore et al. 2008)	Fattore et al. (2009)	Gabhainn and Sixsmith (2005)	Andresen and Fegter (2011)
Support to attain goals				x		
Participation in (un)structured activities				x	x	x
Travel and holidays					x	x
Play					x	x
Place in community	X		X (context)			
Pre-school enrollment	x					
High school diploma	x					
Youth not working, not in school	x					
Bachelor's degree	x					
Voting in Presidential Elections	x					
Supportive neighborhood			x			
Neighborhood support for parenting			x			
Safe neighborhood			x			
Safe school			x			
Emotional/spiritual	X					
Suicide rates	x					
Weekly religious attendance	x					
Religion	x				x	
Subjective well-being		X				
Personal well-being		x				

(continued)

Table A.1 (continued)

	CWI (Land et al. 2001, 2007, 2011)	EU27 (Bradshaw and Richardson 2009)	NSAF – Microdata (Moore et al. 2008)	Fattore et al. (2009)	Gabhainn and Sixsmith (2005)	Andresen and Fegter (2011)
Well-being at school	x				x	x
Self-defined health	x					
Housing and environment		**X**		**X**		
Overcrowding		x				
(safe) environment		x		x		x
Housing problems		x		x		x
Access to physical environments (play)				x		
Self				**X**		
Self-worth, being a good person			x (psychol. health)	x		
Appreciated and respected				x		x
Sense of personal space				x	x	x
Agency				**X**		
Opportunities to effect change				x		x
Participation				x		
Being a good person				**X**		
Positive values that guide behavior				x		
Appropriate responsibilities				x		
Active engagement in community			x (social health)	x		

(continued)

Table A.1 (continued)

	CWI (Land et al. 2001, 2007, 2011)	EU27 (Bradshaw and Richardson 2009)	NSAF – Microdata (Moore et al. 2008)	Fattore et al. (2009)	Gabhainn and Sixsmith (2005)	Andresen and Fegter (2011)
Family context			**X (context)**			
Parental engagement			x			
Parents attend child's activities			x			
Guardian functioning			x			
Home environment			x			

Printed by Printforce, the Netherlands